D1392258

FIRST

Tel: 020 3228 6141
Email: library@slam.nhs.uk
Web: www.slam.nhs.uk/library

birth your way

Sheila Kitzinger

birth your way

A DORLING KINDERSLEY BOOK

Original edition
Editor Lindy Newton
Senior Editor Carolyn Ryden
Art Editors Sally McKay, Sarah Scrutton
Managing Editor Daphne Razazan
Managing Art Editor Anne-Marie Bulat

First published in Great Britain in 1991
by Dorling Kindersley Limited,
9 Henrietta Street, London WC2E 8PS

This revised edition first published in 2002
Design Brightside
Editor Corinne Asghar
Project Art Editor Nicola Rodway
Managing Editor Corinne Roberts
Senior Art Editor Tracey Ward

Copyright © 2001
Dorling Kindersley Limited, London
Text copyright © 2001 Sheila Kitzinger

A CIP catalogue record for this book is
available from the British Library
ISBN 0 7513 0788 2

contents

why birth
without hospital?

Having a baby is one of the most important passages in your life. You feel the child develop and move inside you. In labour you swim with contractions that are like tidal waves sweeping through your body. As you push the baby down, you know the intensity of the birth passion, and then reach out with eager hands to welcome your baby and cradle this new life in your arms. To see love made flesh is to witness a miracle.

birth choices

Whether birth is difficult or easy, painful or pain-free, long-drawn-out or brief, it need not be a medical event. It should never be conducted as if it were no more than a tooth extraction. For childbirth has much deeper significance than the removal of a baby like a decayed molar from a woman's body. The dawning of consciousness in a human being who is opening eyes for the first time on our world is packed with meaning for the mother and father, as it can be for everyone who shares in this greatest adventure of all.

At least, that is how many women see birth. Not all of us, of course. There are women who think too much fuss is made about the birth experience. They simply want it to be painless and over with as soon as possible so that they can get on with their lives. That is a valid point of view. Some women are happy to accept induction, an epidural, and a forceps delivery, or a planned Caesarean section, and feel more secure knowing that childbirth is being managed by a top obstetrician with skills to augment or replace the natural process. I believe that women should be able to have what they choose in childbirth. It is our bodies to which this is happening, and other people should not make decisions for us or make us feel guilty because they would have chosen a different way.

Many women want information that will enable them to make their own decisions and to prepare themselves for an experience in which they participate fully. They know that it is easier to do this on their own ground, in a place to which helpers come as guests. They would like to give birth outside hospital. This may be either in their own home, or in a birth centre in which the rhythms of a labouring woman's body are honoured and waited on, and where birth is noninterventionist and centred on people, instead of on mechanical processes.

"It's the difference between nurses rushing past you in the corridor, in a place where you don't belong, and inviting people into your home, the place that belongs to you."

Hospitals exist where all members of staff share this attitude, but they are few and far between. You need only one person who is out of tune with such ideas, who believes in the aggressive management of labour, who, instead of being client-oriented, sees a woman as a patient who must obey hospital protocols, one person who is anxious and afraid, and who cannot trust women's bodies, for the environment in which birth takes place to be poisoned, and completely unsuitable for the focused concentration and inner confidence that is needed for a good birth.

what is a "good birth"?

A good birth is not just a matter of safety, or of achieving the goal of a live and physically healthy mother and baby. We want birth to be as safe as we can make it, but should not take it for granted that delivery in an operating theatre is necessarily the best way to achieve this. Childbirth has to do with emotions as well as with the sheer mechanics of descent, rotation, and delivery. It is bound to be so, because it is a major transition in the life of the mother, the father, and the whole family.

Everything that happens during a birth influences the way in which a woman perceives herself afterwards. It can affect the relationship between her and the baby, and between both parents and their baby, for years after the actual birth. Women have written to me to seek help with their intensely negative feelings about births that occurred 30 or 40 years earlier, in an attempt to exorcise finally the self-hatred, guilt, and alienation that they experienced from the time of birth onwards.

A good birth is one which the woman looks back on, whatever happened, with satisfaction and fulfilment. Birth can be positive even when, for reasons that cannot be avoided, there is a great deal of physical pain, or sometimes even grieving. I have known a woman give birth to a baby whom she knew had already died. She was nurtured by her partner's loving support right throughout the labour and, mingled with the agony of their loss, the experience was tender, compassionate, and profound.

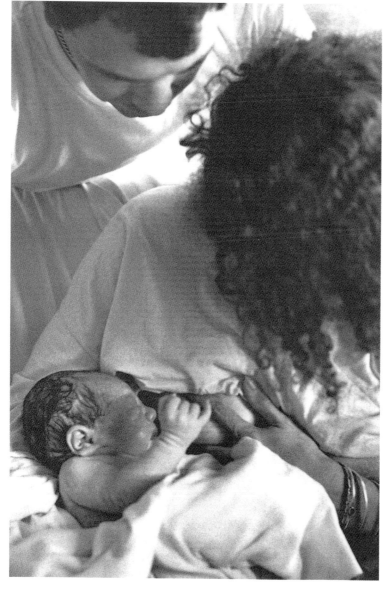

They helped me wrap him up in soft winceyette. He cried a bit. He wasn't particularly interested in the breast but gave it the occasional lick. Then Nick held him while they delivered the placenta without need of synto-metrine. It slithered out five minutes after the birth.

Women who give birth at home believe that this offers the best environment for themselves and their babies. It is far from being a selfish or thoughtless choice. Working towards this kind of birth, and often struggling for it, entails much self-searching, questioning, and negotiation.

Reasons for choosing an out-of-hospital birth Time and again, in discussions I have had with women about their reasons for choosing to give birth at home or in a birth centre rather than in a hospital, the same priorities emerge:

♦ Having a relaxed, peaceful atmosphere for labour and birth.

♦ Feeling the security and comfort of a familiar environment.

♦ Knowing that you are free to be yourself, to do whatever you feel like doing, to move around as you wish, to give birth in any position you choose, and to make any noises that come spontaneously.

♦ Having no interventions, either high-tech obstetric ones, or others that are often done routinely in hospitals, such as artificial rupture of the membranes.

♦ Being able to labour without drugs, and to explore other ways of handling pain.

♦ Knowing that those caring for you are your guests rather than managers, and that you make decisions together, instead of decisions being imposed on you.

♦ Enjoying a relationship of equality with those caring for you.

♦ Having a midwife birth rather than an obstetric delivery.

In the first hour after birth a baby is alert and responsive, so is much more interesting to meet than a bundle in a cot.

♦ Sharing intimately with others who are close to you; enjoying the sense of loving community.
♦ Keeping the family together; having the other children there or close by.
♦ Avoiding an episiotomy and perhaps achieving an intact perineum.
♦ Never being separated from the baby.
♦ Being cared for after birth in a way that is personal and intimate.

Women who feel that they can retain control over what is happening to them during the birth, who understand the options available, and are consulted about what they prefer, are much more likely to experience birth as satisfying than those who are merely at the receiving end of care, however kindly that care. When birth is disempowering, a woman feels degraded, abused, and mutilated.* When birth is empowering, the experience is enriching, her self-confidence is enhanced, and she has a sense of triumph, however difficult the labour was.

I studied women's experiences of epidurals,* and found that women who felt free from any pressure to have one, who were able to obtain the information they wanted and could share in decision-making, were much more likely to feel positive about the birth than those who were under pressure to have an epidural and who felt deprived of autonomy in childbirth. As one woman put it: "I was helpless, treated like a side of meat, moved, examined, and catheterized without consultation as though my labour now belonged to the doctors." In contrast, women for whom the decision to accept the offer of an epidural was one expression of their autonomy in childbirth, rather than a consequence of powerlessness and despair, said, "I felt in control," or "I felt marvellous. I had gone from feeling and behaving like a caged wild animal to being myself, a rational human being." So a central issue in women's birth experiences is that of control: whether we can maintain control over what happens to our bodies, or whether control is taken from us.

To explore all your options about the place of birth, decide on birth at home or in a birth centre, plan ahead to have the kind of birth you want in an environment which you control yourself, to have people you love around you whenever you want, take personal responsibility, and prepare together with your caregivers for the best possible experience in an out-of-hospital setting – this is empowering.

what's wrong with hospitals?

One reason why you may be considering birth outside hospital is that you have heard from other women about their unhappy experiences, have visited the hospital and did not like the atmosphere, or have already had a hospital birth and are determined not to repeat the experience. The same hospital that offers superb care to people who are ill may provide an environment for childbirth that introduces unnecessary risks, obstructs the normal process, and inculcates in women who are giving birth anxiety, dependency, fear, and loss of self-confidence.

the hospital system

The maternity hospitals of the 18th and 19th centuries were created as charity institutions for poor women who had nowhere else to go and for unmarried women bearing their babies in shame. Other women gave birth at home. These institutions provided raw material for obstetric practice, and women were used to demonstrate obstetrics and gynaecology to medical students. They were guinea pigs for research too. The first experiments for artificially inducing labour were conducted on poor women who could not afford doctors' fees and who entered hospital as clinic patients.

In the United States, poor women without health insurance still provide a pool of patients on whom students can learn. In Britain women having babies in teaching hospitals may find medical students grouped round the bed, and may never discover that the doctor who laboriously stitched an episiotomy was a house officer learning how to do it for the first time.

Following the Second World War, the British National Health Service made medical care accessible to all without need to worry about payment. Many other European countries created social security and health care systems funded by tax-payers, based on the policy that health care is a national responsibility.

With the creation of the National Health Service there came government health policies about childbirth and where it should take place. The decision was made that there should be sufficient beds for all women to have their babies in hospital, and birth became more and more medicalized. This was happening at a time when the standard of living was rising fast. A generation of British children had grown up who had benefited from the simple, good nutrition of the war years – wholemeal bread, orange juice, milk, few fats, little meat, and high consumption of vegetables. People were healthier than ever before. As a result, women were more likely to be fit during their pregnancy, did not suffer from anaemia, and did not think of pregnancy as an illness. Babies were born healthier, and the perinatal mortality rate – the death of babies at and immediately after birth – dropped progressively, so that now it is at an all time low of 8 per 1,000 births.

Obstetricians claim that this is due to better obstetric services, and to the policy of hospital birth for all. Yet still today women who are at the bottom of the social scale, whose partners are manual workers or who are unemployed, are twice as likely to have a baby who dies as middle class women. Social differences – education, general health, access to information, housing conditions, nutrition, attitudes to smoking, and ease of communication between caregivers and patients – have a powerful effect on the perinatal mortality rate. Babies die and women suffer in childbirth and afterwards because of poverty and neglect.

Sophisticated equipment, modern, high-technology machines, anaesthetists and doctors with surgical skills are available only in hospital, of course. This equipment and these skills can be life-saving – for a small minority of babies. But increasingly researchers are asking whether the intervention that takes place, often routinely, in many hospital births may not be hazardous. Most of these techniques have been introduced without adequate research. The question is whether procedures such as induction of labour, stimulation of the uterus with drugs once labour has started, artificial rupture of the membranes, the use of large quantities of pain-killing drugs, and continuous electronic monitoring of the fetus may not be harmful for mothers and babies if they take place as a matter of routine and are not used selectively.

Hospital ritual

The trouble is that almost every woman going into hospital today finds that procedures she does not wish to have are mandatory because of hospital protocols about care and rules laid down by obstetricians.

♦ Your waters may be broken artificially when the cervix is 3-4 cm dilated.

♦ If your cervix does not dilate by 1 cm per hour labour may be speeded up. This entails an intravenous drip in the arm and a uterine stimulant dripped into your bloodstream.

♦ You may be under pressure to have drugs for pain relief that you do not want.

"They just told me what they were going to do. They never asked what I wanted."

♦ You may be allowed only two hours, an hour and a half, an hour, or even 45 minutes, to deliver following full dilatation – before being given a forceps delivery or vacuum extraction.

There are more subtle interventions too – things that affect the atmosphere in which birth takes place and the attitudes of everyone participating. They include:

♦ Having to put on a hospital gown.

♦ Being put to bed as if you were ill.

♦ Not being able to eat and drink when you want to.

♦ Constant checking of the progress of labour against the clock.

♦ Different members of staff coming and going.

♦ Having no privacy and being surrounded by strangers who talk over you and about you, rather than to you.

♦ Being treated like an irresponsible child.

In some hospitals the whole emphasis is on pathology – detecting things that might go wrong – instead of on supporting the spontaneous flow of labour.

These interventions can lead to a massive loss of confidence in a woman. She is expected to be passive and obedient – a "good patient". She comes to distrust her body. She may feel alienated from everything that is happening to her, and this although caregivers are trying to be kind. They may be unaware of how she is feeling and of the distress that is bottled up inside her, to emerge only later, days, weeks, or months after the baby is born. She is likely to believe that all her negative emotions about the birth, and the way in which it is replayed over and over again in her mind, and sometimes too, the hostility that bursts out towards her baby, are her own fault, and she feels terribly guilty.

new developments

Astonishing changes in obstetrics and in women's attitudes to childbirth occurred from the 70s and on through the 90s. A new partnership between obstetrics and electronic engineering opened up windows on the womb with ultrasound; technological innovations made birth more complicated, compelling the mother to be a passive patient; and birth was seen by obstetricians as a medical event that could take place only in an intensive care setting equipped to meet all possible disasters. At the same time, women have been clamouring for care that is more personal, more sensitive to their needs, in an environment in which they can be in tune with the spontaneous psycho-biological processes of birth and the creative energy pouring through their bodies.

"It isn't a matter of what it looks like. The hospital birthing rooms are all chintzy. But the staff decide what you do and when you do it. They're in control. I don't want to be 'managed' by anybody."

The result has been, on the one hand, more and more obstetric intervention and, on the other, a reformation movement in which women are rediscovering the value of small-scale, low-tech birthplaces. They are increasingly seeking alternative settings such as birth centres and birth rooms, and even, in spite of intense opposition from the medical system, making the decision to give birth in their own homes.

"Birth is birth, not pain. Closing my eyes I can imagine the birth of mountains to describe the forces at work in my body."

Women walk about throughout the first stage of labour and midwives – and more rarely obstetricians – help mothers get into any position in which it is comfortable for them to give birth. Birth plans have been widely introduced. Women are asked what they would like to do and have done during their labour, and caregivers are listening more to their patients, and recording their wishes in the case-notes. All these developments are to be warmly welcomed. We are making progress.

One question to resolve is, "Will birth in this place be both safe and empowering for me as a woman?"

Even so, hospitals are institutions – and often very large, complex, bureaucratic, and hierarchically organized institutions. They have to be managed so that the different parts of the whole structure can work together efficiently. Under these circumstances it is easy to abrogate responsibility and for an individual's main concern to be to oil the wheels of the system and make it run smoothly. It is not surprising that women's needs and wishes are often ignored or trivialized. Hospitals would function much more efficiently if there were no patients.

"The best thing about it was being at home and with my family."

In hospital patients may be allowed choice, but they have no real power. The territory belongs to the hospital management. When I analysed the words used by 40 women who had given birth at home and compared their accounts with 40 others by women who all delivered vaginally in hospital, I found that many of those in hospital used words such as "allowed" or "let me", but that no home birth mothers used these words. Although many hospital birth mothers felt very positive about their experience, they did not have the same sense of being able to control what happened to them.

"Breathing slowly, feeling the pain with satisfaction and pleasure, in my own room at peace."

Pain is never as simple as just having a 'high' or 'low' pain threshold. It always has a meaning. It does not exist in a vacuum. It rouses personal memories of being in pain, and of witnessing other people's pain. The way we approach pain may be affected by other women's descriptions of their labours, as well as birth images in the media, and often half-forgotten childhood memories, too.

It may help if you think how do you usually handle pain? Not only labour pain, but other kinds, too. If you immediately reach for some capsules to deaden it, home birth may not be right for you. If you think about what *causes* the pain, and as a result try to reduce the pressures you are under, change what you eat, adjust your posture and the way you move, and especially if you have discovered how relaxation, breathing and focused concentration can help you handle pain, home birth may be a good choice.

"The head crowned and stayed as the contraction went off and whoa! What a stretch! I had to pant as I waited for the next contraction and wondered if I would split open! Bobbie passed me a mirror and I shook my head, trying to stay focused. Then quickly my body gave another push and out came the head."

Home birth works best for women who want to *cope* with pain, rather than hand the pain over to be reduced or eradicated by professionals.

Labour pain is different from the pain of injury. It is caused by muscles stretching, pressure against nerves, and your body opening. It is similar to menstrual pain, but much more intense. It comes in waves. This rhythm means that there is a rest period between each contraction. As your cervix dilates progressively these rest periods become very short. There is just sufficient time in which to breathe out, drop shoulders, relax, and centre yourself, before the next wave rushes over you.

The *meaning* of birth pain is different from the pain of, say, tooth or earache, broken bones or colic. It is the pain of creative activity.

In a labour that is going well each contraction starts gently, builds up in a grand crescendo to a peak, and then fades away. It is pain with a purpose – *positive* pain.

This is not to say that birth pain is easy to bear. For many women it is the hardest pain they have ever experienced. It has been rated among the most severe pain ever known.* Yet it is profoundly affected by what is going on in your mind and the attitudes of whoever is helping you.

Pain is a private experience. No-one can tell you that their pain is more or less than yours. This is why it is difficult to evaluate it and place it on a scale of 0–10. It all depends on the significance that the pain has in terms of your life, your relationships and the surroundings.

"I looked down to see her on the floor, a wriggling, slithering little body with all her rolls of loose skin, pale and brown stained, hair plastered onto her head. I said "hello, my darling, it's OK" and put my hands down to pick her up."

It is difficult for anyone who has had a distressing labour to understand how other women can enjoy giving birth. It seems to some women that when others talk about the joy of birth, and of triumphantly riding the waves of contractions, they must be romanticising or telling lies. A woman who, for example, relies on getting an epidural as soon as she turns up at the hospital, but is denied one because the anaesthetist is not available, or the midwife considers it too late in labour to give it, and that it would lead to an unnecessary operative delivery, is likely to feel extreme and uncontrollable pain. She also feels anger that may be turned on to those who denied her the pain relief she wanted and on to other women who look back on their labours with satisfaction and delight. It is not hard to understand why this happens. This does not rule out the fact that it is possible to relish the birth experience, in the right environment, and with the right people in attendance. This is why women choose home birth. They want to be on their own territory.

"I had just climbed Annapurna and accepted the Nobel prize all in the course of little more than day."

Research reveals that women who are not looking forward to the baby suffer more pain than those who are eager to have the baby. When a partner is negative about or hostile to a pregnancy this may lead to birth being more painful too.*

When a woman is very anxious towards the end of pregnancy she tends to feel more pain in labour than one who is happy, and if she *expects* to feel a lot of pain, she really experiences more, probably because she is tense and already in a state of psycho-physiological 'fight or flight'.* And when a woman is isolated and alone during the first stage of labour everything becomes more painful.*

the effects of stress

Labour is stressful for most women, even in an out-of-hospital setting where they feel safe, confident, and among friends. In hospital, environmental stress is added to this psychological stress.

Birth in hospital is often very stressful because a woman finds herself in a strange place; she has to cope with a number of different professionals who care for her during labour, and the emphasis is on things that may go wrong. It is not simply a matter of physical pain. This added stress combines with the stress from the pain.

"She was so slippery and I was now shaking uncontrollably so Bobbie helped her into my arms and I lay back and held her on my tummy. I could hardly hold her for shaking and her squirming and slipperiness, but there she was, and I was trying to calm us both."

Distress tends to interfere with the efficiency of uterine action, and labour slows down or the woman is unable to push her baby out. Because it interferes with the physiology of birth, this excessive stress may affect the condition of the baby both before and after the birth.

When under stress our bodies produce catecholamines, or "stress hormones", the best-known of which are adrenalin and nonadrenalin. This is normal and advantageous under most circumstances, because cathecholamines help the body adjust to stress. But if stress is excessive, or goes on too long, the body exhausts its resources.

When catecholamine levels rise abnormally in a woman in labour, her uterus contracts less efficiently, contractions become weaker or spasmodic, dilatation of the cervix is slower, and labour longer.*

"Though stinging, trembling and in shock, I was ecstatic. I couldn't believe it. Here was that being I'd been talking to all those months, longing to hold in my arms. I gave thanks for our safe delivery and whispered "We did it. We're safe. I love you"."

Sometimes the uterus stops contracting for a while. This often occurs when she first arrives in hospital, even when contractions have been strong and regular at home. The rise in catecholamine levels has the effect of making her more anxious, which also means that she feels more pain. This further increases catecholamine levels. It is a vicious circle.

However, when there is no added stress, the hard work of labour, the mother's excitement, the mobilization of her energy to meet the challenge of contractions as they get stronger, longer, and closer together, are good for the baby. The fetus also makes its own catecholamines.

When catecholamines are at a normal level, they:
♦ Stimulate production of prostaglandins and oxygen uptake.
♦ Protect the baby from the effects of reduced flow of blood through the placenta at the height of contractions.
♦ Cause blood to be shunted from near the skin surface to the baby's vital organs – the heart, brain, and liver.

They help the baby adjust to life outside the uterus by:
♦ Facilitating absorption of liquid in the lungs.
♦ Enabling the baby to generate its own heat.
♦ Producing the alert, attentive state that helps parents fall in love with their baby.

But if catecholamines are pushed above this physiological level when the mother is under great stress during labour:
♦ Less oxygenated blood flows to the uterus and through the placenta to the baby.
♦ The baby compensates by producing catecholamines, with resulting fetal heart irregularities.

> **A doctor:**
> "I have just had my first baby at home. It was an incredible experience – the equivalent of climbing Mount Everest."

Very high catecholamine levels may lead to problems for the newborn baby too:
♦ Breathing difficulties.
♦ Difficulty in regulating his temperature.
♦ Reduction in plasma volume (the liquid part of blood).
♦ Metabolic acidosis (chemical imbalance in the blood).
♦ Jaundice (excess bile pigment in blood).
♦ Even sometimes necrotizing enterocolitis (diarrhoea with blood in the faeces).

Obstetric anaesthetists who are concerned about the effect of high catecholamine levels on babies have responded by recommending that small hospitals should be closed, all women admitted to large regional hospitals, and as many offered epidural anaesthesia as the epidural service can handle.* It is true that an epidural can provide blessed relief when a woman is in uncontrollable pain. But often the pain is actually caused by the way she is being treated. The hospital environment, with its rules, tests, and the constant threat of obstetric intervention, is pushing up both the mother's catecholamine levels and those of her baby.

why not hospital?

Hospitals are often dangerous places in which to give birth. It is usually taken for granted that they must be safe because they have the equipment and skilled staff to deal with medical emergencies. But sometimes they are the cause of these emergencies in the first place. Many interventions that take place routinely in hospital birth are iatrogenic. That is, they result in illness produced by doctors.

Induction

This is the most frequent reason for women to be transferred from home to hospital before labour starts.

An obstetrician:

"When a woman is at home and you want to intervene, it forces you to think whether it's really necessary. The very ease with which interventions take place in hospital increases the risk of them being performed unnecessarily."

Rates of induction vary widely in different countries, and between different obstetricians. Women often do not even know why their labours are being induced. It is the doctor's decision, and the mother is expected to go along with it for the sake of her baby. But induction is not always successful. It is most likely to succeed if a woman's cervix is ripe. Ripeness is assessed by the 'Bishop score'. Only if that exceeds 8 are the chances of success the same as if labour starts spontaneously.

The risks of induction*
♦ Induction does not always work. Failed induction leads to Caesarean section.
♦ If the baby's head is not well down and membranes are ruptured artificially the first rush of amniotic fluid may bring the cord down and deprive the baby of oxygen.
♦ Rupture of the membranes can cause infection.
♦ An induced labour is often fast and furious, so it is more painful than one that starts naturally. In my own study of some women's experiences of induced labour* I found that when women whose second labour was induced compared this with the previous labour which had not been induced,

Induction

Q **Why are labours induced?**

Inductions, like other interventions, can be useful in selected situations. If a woman has pre-eclampsia, for example, and her blood pressure is dangerously high, the placenta may fail to support the baby, so it may be safer to deliver early. A diabetic woman's baby tends to grow very large and, though preterm, it is safer to deliver early.

Q **Are there any other reasons?**

A doctor may want to induce if you go two weeks, ten days, or even a few days, past your due date. Some like to induce at term – on or around the expected date, or even a week early – on the grounds that "this is a very precious baby", especially with an older mother. There are women who are fed up with being pregnant or who prefer to know exactly when the birth will be, and who welcome induction for this reason. Inductions for convenience are often disguised as medically indicated.

Q **How is labour induced?**

Induction is done in one, or a combination, of three ways: synthetic oxytocin is introduced into your bloodstream. Prostaglandin in the form of a gel is placed in your cervix. Amniotomy is performed – the water bubble in which the baby lies is broken with an instrument resembling a crochet hook or small forceps.

Q **Will I still be able to have an active birth?**

No. It is impossible to move freely, or sometimes even to change position in bed with ease. You have an intravenous drip in your arm, a blood pressure cuff encircling your upper arm, a catheter in your bladder, an electrode screwed or clipped into the baby's scalp to record its

heartbeat, and if you have an epidural, a plastic tube stuck in your back and snaking up to your shoulder, where it is fixed with sticky tape so that the epidural can be topped up.

Q **What other interventions might there be?**

Because induction makes labour more painful it is often given in a package deal with epidural anaesthesia. Then other interventions may take place which add new risks with a knock-on effect. Having a catheter inserted in your bladder increases the risk of infection, for example. Labour is always monitored electronically when induction takes place. This increases the chance of an operative vaginal delivery or a Caesarean.

two-thirds of them said that the second labour was more painful, though as a rule second labours are less painful.

♦ Being immobilized makes it more likely that dilatation is slow, and so the drip is turned up and more artificial oxytocin is fed into the bloodstream. Large quantities of fluid may produce water intoxication. A woman who drinks as much fluid as she wants during labour does not take too much. But, if fluids are introduced through an intravenous drip, her metabolism is altered, and, if she receives an excessive quantity, she may suffer convulsions. When oxytocin is being dripped into a woman's bloodstream in addition to glucose solution, she is further at risk of water intoxication.

"The pain was shocking – double-peaked contractions that lasted almost two minutes."

♦ Occasionally the uterus becomes hypertonic. That is, it clamps down on the baby with strong contractions lasting two minutes or longer, and this reduces the flow of blood. In normal labour contractions squeeze the baby as if it were being hugged tightly. Blood flow is lessened at the height of contractions, but increased as each one finishes. In induced labour there is a risk that this rhythm is lost and that the uterus goes into spasm. The result is that the baby's heartbeat becomes either very fast – tachycardia – or slow – bradycardia. At birth the baby may need resuscitation and be taken to the special care nursery for observation.

♦ Hyperstimulation of the uterus sometimes results in uterine rupture, especially in women who have had babies before.

♦ There is increased risk of amniotic fluid embolism – a bubble of fluid entering the mother's circulation.

At home or in a birth centre labour is not induced. This is because it is recognized that induction brings risks and may entail other forms of intervention, including drugs for pain relief and an assisted delivery. These are incompatible with care outside hospital. Having a baby at home is one way of ruling out entirely a whole category of risks that starts with induction, escalates with pain-killing drugs, and peaks when uterine stimulants are stepped up because drugs have made contractions weaker or erratic.

Active management

In many hospitals today labours are managed "actively". That is, the obstetrician takes charge, with the aim of making labour conform to a norm. A typical pattern is that it should not last longer than 12 hours, dilatation should take place by at least 1 cm an hour, and delivery must occur within one hour of full dilatation.

If a labour is not conforming to this model, intravenous oxytocin is used to stimulate the uterus to greater activity, or delivery is completed with forceps, vacuum extraction, or Caesarean section.* Active management was first introduced in Dublin, where the emphasis is on a short, snappy labour, and also on one-to-one nurse care. (For some reason the Irish obstetricians who started this system ignore midwives and talk about "nurses" instead.) They call it "military efficiency with a human face".* The original plan was that no fathers should be present, epidurals would rarely be given, and pethidine only in small doses. "The time of delivery is stated to within 30 minutes: a woman is told at noon that her baby is expected at four o'clock in the afternoon, give or take half an hour."* Women must labour silently: "A woman owes it to herself, to her husband, and to her child, and to every other woman *who may be unfortunate enough to labour at the same time* [my italics], to be well-briefed in this matter. The disruptive effect of one disorganized and frightened woman in a delivery unit extends far beyond her own comfort and safety, and there should be no hesitation in telling her so."

"They ruptured my membranes, set up a glucose drip, and put a scalp electrode on the baby's head. I felt trapped. Then they added syntocinon to the drip and gave me pethidine."

Mothers have a duty also to those who care for them during labour: "It should be clearly understood that nurses must not be expected to submit to the sometimes outrageous conduct of perfectly healthy women who cannot be persuaded to behave with dignity and purpose during the most important hours of their lives – nor should nurses be held responsible in any way for the degrading scenes which occasionally result."* So, when a woman pleads for pain-killers, weeps in terror, or screams out in agony, these obstetricians consider that it is her fault.

"I had an intravenous drip and was strapped up to two fetal monitors. I longed to get upright, but it was impossible."

The use of oxytocin to augment a labour that has already started is not without risk. Just as when it is used for induction, labour is more painful for the mother, there may be hyperstimulation of the uterus, and the baby may become short of oxygen. This is why obstetricians in Dublin do not advise the use of oxytocin in multigravidae (women who have already had babies). Elsewhere, however, active management may include the routine speeding up of labour, even when the problem is not, in fact, uterine "inefficiency" but disproportion – that is, when the baby cannot pass through the mother's pelvis. Then the uterus may rupture (the muscle tears). The baby may be short of oxygen – hypoxia; in some cases the baby may turn out to have cerebral palsy as a result, and occasionally the mother's pelvis may even be fractured.*

"I was given oxytocin with no explanation. They told my husband, 'She's being a bit slow.' It was a very shocking experience."

When you give birth in territory which you control, instead of management protocols dictating how labour should be conducted, you are yourself the active birth-giver. This is the fundamental difference between birth in hospital and birth at home or in the kind of birth centre where the power is yours, not the doctor's.

Electronic fetal monitoring

Many obstetricians believe that continuous electronic fetal monitoring should be employed in all labours "just in case". In hospital, monitoring is done either from the time a woman is admitted until she delivers, or a "strip" print-out is taken for about an hour after she is admitted and, if all is well, taken again only if further information is required later in the labour.

There is marked disagreement between obstetricians about what ought to be done when the print-out from the monitor is different from what would normally be expected. When four experienced

"Everything was just "done" to me. I wasn't consulted about anything and it was all out of my control."

obstetricians studied the same fetal heart traces and were asked whether they would deliver immediately, they agreed in only one out of five cases.* Nearly two years later these obstetricians were shown the same traces again and asked what they would do. In one out of five cases they assessed them differently from the time before.

There is no evidence that electronic fetal monitoring saves babies' lives or that the condition of babies at birth has anything to do with whether or not they had electronic monitoring during labour.* It has been discovered, however, that when babies are monitored they are less likely to have neonatal seizures.* This might be a very important finding, except that further studies have revealed that these seizures are not linked with any long-term problems.*

Risks of electronic monitoring At first glance it might look as if this particular piece of high technology could do nothing but good. But the trouble is that electronic fetal monitoring itself causes problems and introduces its own risks.

♦ If monitoring is to be employed safely, caregivers must know how to use it and understand how to interpret the information correctly. This is not always the case. Sometimes the monitor picks up the mother's heartbeat rather than the baby's, for example. Since the baby's heart is normally about twice as fast as hers, it then appears as if there is fetal bradycardia. Unnecessary intervention takes place, and the baby may be delivered by forceps or Caesarean section.*

♦ Sometimes the opposite happens: caregivers are lulled into false security when a woman is wired up to a monitor and no one bothers to check the print-out regularly or looks at the whole pattern of her labour. The monitor cannot give birth. Only the woman can do that. The monitor records data, and what is done or not done then depends on the skills of the caregivers.

♦ Although some monitors work with radio waves – telemetry – and allow a woman to walk about, the use of most monitors means that she must stay in one place, either strapped up tightly with belts around her abdomen or wired up with a pin stuck in the baby's head. This immobilization causes unnecessary pain and may slow down contractions and make them weaker, so that dilatation is slower. Sometimes labour becomes so slow that the decision is made to augment it with an oxytocin intravenous drip.

> "They put me on an oxytocin drip against my will. I was left with a student who read the paper and totally ignored me."

♦ A woman is often told to lie still so that the print-out is clear.* If she is lying on her back, not only does she get backache, but there is a danger of compression of her aorta – the large blood vessel in the lower part of her body – by her heavy uterus, with a resulting slow down in the flow of blood back to her heart. She becomes sick, dizzy, faint, and may even black out. This deprives the baby of oxygen too. The monitor then spills out ominous traces in the fetal heart-rate, recording information about a situation which it was responsible for creating in the first place.

♦ When there are staff shortages, or when staff do not understand the importance of being centred on the woman and creating a calm, loving atmosphere, a partner is often told to keep an eye on the monitor, or a midwife pops in at intervals, studies the print-out, says a cheery word to the mother, and disappears again. Attention turns to the electronic equipment rather than being focused on the woman's needs, and she loses emotional support. Even with her partner close beside her, a woman may then be isolated. An electronic monitor cannot take the place of human caring and understanding. Mind and body are not two separate, distinct systems in childbirth. A woman's body works best when she is confident, secure, emotionally supported, and on her own ground.

♦ An electrode can be fixed on the baby's head only after the membranes have ruptured. If this has not occurred spontaneously in early labour, an amniotomy is performed, usually at 3 or 4 cm dilatation. When there is no interference, membranes usually do not rupture at the beginning of labour, but at the very end of the first stage. Artificial rupture of the membranes interferes with the sterile environment in which the baby is contained and may result in infection. It also removes the protection provided by the water bubble which normally cushions the baby and its cord and placenta against excessive pressure. The result is that blood flow may be impeded. The monitor then demonstrates that the baby is in trouble, but it was the amniotomy to put the electrode on the baby's head that was responsible for the stress to the baby.

♦ Some doctors are experimenting with ways of fixing electrodes using strong suction or glue so that they do not have to harpoon the baby, but they have not yet succeeded in producing a viable alternative to scalp clips or screws. When a baby's scalp is penetrated by the hook or spiral screw, the scalp may be damaged when removing it.* Sometimes there is a bald patch and hair never grows there, or an abscess forms, which has to be treated with antibiotics.*

♦ In most hospitals the introduction of electronic fetal monitoring immediately pushes the Caesarean section rate up at least three-fold. After the equipment has been in use for some time, staff relax a bit and the rate drops again. But in industrialized countries worldwide there is a steady increase in Caesareans, which can be attributed partly to electronic monitoring. Caesarean section is riskier for women than vaginal birth. Five times as many women die after a Caesarean than after a vaginal birth (50 compared with 10 per 100,000 deliveries), and there is a much increased risk of infection and other postpartum problems.*

♦ Information that the fetal monitor provides bears little or no relation to the baby's condition at birth. Too little is known about normal variations in the fetal heart-rate to warrant intervention only on the basis of a suspicious trace on an electronic monitor.

♦ Many monitors don't work well all the time. Women say that they were told: "Oh, don't take any notice of that. It isn't working properly," or a partner is advised to kick the machine when a light starts flashing because "it's always doing that. It doesn't mean anything." Yet the rule is that the woman must be attached to a monitor, even though it is not providing accurate information. This can be a very bewildering and frightening experience. Under these circumstances the monitor is worse than useless. It is actually dangerous.

Intermittent monitoring

The older way of monitoring the condition of the baby during labour was to listen to its heart intermittently through a trumpet-shaped fetal stethoscope.

The accuracy of this method depends on how often and when it is done. It is important to know whether the fetal heart is picking up regularly after contractions. The baby who is over-stressed is usually the one whose heart speeds up a lot – above 160 beats a minute – or slows down below 120 beats a minute with contractions, and stays high or low in the space between contractions. When the heart slows down at the peak of contractions, a perfectly natural occurrence, it is called early (or variable) deceleration. When the heart stays slow afterwards, it is a late deceleration. It is late decelerations that are worrying. If a baby is in real trouble, there are few or no variations in heart-rate. The trace is flat.

A doctor:
"I did a home birth and had for the first time a feeling of confidence because it was just happening. Any medical intervention would have been entirely inappropriate."

So if a fetal stethoscope is the method of choice, it should be used at the end of every cluster of strong contractions in the late first stage, and more often in the second stage, the times in labour when contractions may be most stressful for the baby. Having a fetal stethoscope poked at you just as a contraction ends can be uncomfortable and irritating. Many women and midwives prefer a newer intermittent method of monitoring which uses Doppler ultrasound in the form of a hand-held sonic aid. This is a camera-sized instrument with a disc like a small microphone which is held over the baby's heart, registers the beats, and translates these into an audible signal – like galloping horses.

This method provides no permanent record of the heart-rate in the form of a printed trace, and this could be a disadvantage from the point of view of obstetricians anxious about possible litigation after the birth. However, litigation is very unlikely after a birth that has taken place, by the woman's choice, out of hospital, and without obstetric intervention.

So high-tech gadgets may be useful, but only those that do not intrude on your ability to tune in to your body and to the power that wells up inside you, on the full tide of which your baby is brought to birth.

Pain-relieving drugs

One reason why women seek home birth is that they hope to have a drug-free labour. All anaesthetic and analgesic drugs given to the mother cross the placenta to the fetus. I have heard an obstetric anaesthetist describe the placenta as "a sump for drugs". Drug transfer is flow dependent. Fetal plasma has a lower pH than maternal plasma, so the drug concentrates in the fetus. Pethidine, for example, is a weak analgesic but a strong respiratory depressant. After a single dose there is a higher concentration in the fetus than in the mother, and it can be detected in the newborn baby for 62 hours.

Epidurals

An epidural can give blessed relief from pain and it does not produce respiratory depression. When it is performed by an experienced anaesthetist it is usually safe. But it may have side-effects for the mother and the baby. Fifteen percent of mothers and babies develop fever during labour, for example. The baby may be taken to the special care nursery for tests to discover if it is suffering from septicaemia.

Another thing that may happen is that the mother's blood pressure drops suddenly when the epidural is given. This reduces the oxygen passing to the baby. So other drugs have to be available to raise her blood pressure again. Delivery may be by forceps or ventouse (vacuum extraction) because the tone of the pelvic floor muscles is lost, the head gets stuck in the wrong position, and the mother cannot push the baby out. The vaginal operative delivery rate is four times higher than when a woman does not have an epidural, and the Caesarean rate is twice as high. Paralysis is extremely rare.*

The rushed second stage

Clock-watched labours are the rule in hospitals. When women describe their labours in hospital, they often refer to the time. They say things like:

"My induction was well-timed to fit into working hours," "The pupil midwife told me to watch the clock and time contractions," or "The baby was posterior, and the midwife said they'd give me a few hours to see what happened." When women give birth at home, they talk about meal-times, sunrise, sunlight pouring in through the window, trees tossing in the wind, birds singing, in sunset and night-time, but they do not usually relate everything that occured in labour to the clock.

In my own study of the language women used in describing 40 home and 40 hospital births, three-quarters of home birth mothers said that they enjoyed not being hurried and knowing that they had plenty of time.* Only four hospital birth mothers made similar statements.

In hospital the clock is master, marking the distinction between the normal and the abnormal, the labour that can be allowed to proceed without obstetric intervention and the labour that calls for immediate intervention.

Doctors and midwives who attend home births usually know how to watch and wait. They realize that the uterus works most effectively if a woman is in an upright or semi-upright position and can alter her position when she wants. They know that moving around can often change malposition or malpresentation. They are aware that anxiety and fear can make it harder for a woman to open her body and push her baby out. If she is not wasting energy trying to push, and pushes only when she wants to, and for only as long as she wants to, she can work with her body, instead of fighting against it.

"The doctor gave me 20 minutes to push while she got the forceps ready. It was harrowing."

A second stage in which you are harried and hurried is bound to be an anxious and panic-inducing ordeal. In hospital, women are often coaxed or commanded to push, and instructed to hold each breath and push as hard as they possibly can, because of the time limit on the second stage.

In British hospitals, women having their first babies (primiparae) are usually allowed only one hour from full dilation to delivery. Some obstetricians consider that this is far too long, and limit first-time mothers to 45 minutes or even half an hour, and multiparae to 20 minutes.*

There is no evidence that reducing the length of the second stage makes labour any safer, prevents baby deaths, or produces healthier babies.* If a baby is too large to come through the mother's pelvis, there are many clinical signs. These include the head staying high, lack of progress, fetal heart arrhythmia, and late decelerations that indicate this – not the length of the second stage alone.

The mother is often encouraged to hold her breath over prolonged periods when pushing, and this can be dangerous, because it may reduce the baby's oxygen.* One problem in many hospitals is that the second stage is reckoned to start with full dilatation of the cervix. Frequent vaginal examinations result in full dilatation being assessed and noted on the case record or partogram (labour chart) immediately it is reached, or even sometimes before this. The second stage is then timed from that point. But the woman may not yet want to push. This is natural. If the baby's head is not pressing against your pelvic floor muscles, you have no spontaneous desire to push, since this is a reflex stimulated when there is pressure against nerve endings in the pelvic floor.

From then it is a race to the finishing post. The woman may be bullied in an effort to get the baby born before the obstetrician must be called, and delivery completed with episiotomy and forceps or vacuum extraction, or a Caesarean section.

Episiotomy

You are much more likely to have an episiotomy – a cut in the vagina which is made to enlarge the birth opening – if you have your baby in a hospital than you are if you give birth at home or in a midwife-led birth centre.

Episiotomy rates vary widely between countries, and even between hospitals and different obstetricians in the same hospital. In some countries as many as nine out of ten women receive an episiotomy.* Some obstetricians believe that all first-time mothers should have an episiotomy.

They may believe, too, that any woman who has had an episiotomy should have one with the next delivery, because scar tissue must be present that will not stretch to let the baby out easily. The result is that everyone has an episiotomy except those who deliver too fast to have one.

Pros and cons of episiotomy Episiotomy is performed with the aim of saving the baby from being "battered" against the mother's pelvic floor, to prevent damage to these muscles, to avoid injury to her anus, to prevent later stress incontinence (leaking of urine), and to achieve better healing than after laceration with "a nice clean cut that is easier to sew up than a nasty, jagged tear". There is no evidence that episiotomy does any of these things.* Even if it did not matter what happened to the mother, and if episiotomies were performed for the baby's sake alone, the claim that episiotomy protects the baby's head, or produces a baby in better condition, is not supported by the evidence.*

Because obstetricians make rules as to how long their patients may be in the second stage, midwives and junior doctors delivering babies with no obstetrician present perform episiotomies to hasten delivery if they come up against that time limit.*

Although occasionally the baby's head can be nicked by scissors, the hazards of episiotomy generally concern the mother, not the baby, in a number of ways:

♦ Having an episiotomy is often acutely painful. If it is performed at the height of a contraction when the perineum is stretched and bulging, a woman may not feel it. But, because of possible damage to the baby's head, in hospitals there are rules about it being done only between contractions. A local anaesthetic is often – not always – given first, but this itself hurts in a very sensitive place, and in many hospitals staff do not wait the three or four minutes necessary for the perineum to be absolutely numb before cutting.*

♦ Repair of an episiotomy is often painful, too. The wound must be sutured carefully, correctly aligning damaged tissues. Inadequate local anaesthesia may be used, or one part not numbed at all, or the person doing the suturing may not wait for the anaesthetic to take effect. So perineal repair is for some women more painful than anything they experienced during the birth – much more painful than contractions or the delivery.

♦ The area is often bruised. This may be because the baby's head has been bumping against it, but the most severe bruising results from an episiotomy made too early, before the head is on the perineum. This is regular practice in some hospitals, on the grounds that in this way any stress caused by the baby's head is prevented. The scissors used may be blunt, so that they crush as well as cut the tissues, and extensive bruising results then, too.

♦ Blood loss with episiotomy may cause anaemia and make a woman feel very weak and tired, and this at a time when she wants to be alert to get to know her newborn baby. The combination of exhaustion and pain is very demoralizing and makes a frightening start to motherhood.

♦ Many episiotomy wounds become infected, and sometimes a perineal abscess results. This is terribly painful. Infection is more common in hospital than at home, and many hospital bacteria are now penicillin resistant. Infection delays healing and, when the wound does at last heal, there may be scar tissue.

♦ Although episiotomies are performed in the theory that to make a deliberate cut prevents a tear into the anus and rectum, a third-degree laceration (fourth-degree in the USA), this occurs more often when an episiotomy has been performed than when a tear occurs naturally. A small proportion of women have an episiotomy plus a laceration, because the cut has then gone on to tear. The intricate embroidery that has to be done when this happens may entail general anaesthesia and can take a long time. The woman is in far more pain afterwards than after a second-degree laceration.*

♦ In the week after a woman's perineum has been sutured, as healing takes place, she is likely to be in constant discomfort, and in pain when she empties her bladder or bowels, walks, shifts position in bed, or lifts and feeds her baby. Women on postnatal wards shuffle around, bent forward, knees together, trying to cope with this pain. The second, third, and fourth days are often the worst, and then things become easier. The pain after a first-degree tear – a nick in the skin only – is much less than that after an episiotomy, which corresponds to a second-degree tear, cutting into muscle.*

The lasting effects

Discomfort often lasts for some months, with a knot of scar tissue at the lower end of the vagina which may be too painful to touch. At three months postpartum a large percentage of women still have pain some of the time: if they sit down on a hard chair without thinking, wear trousers that are tight on the crotch, stand too long, or move carelessly. Women whose periods have returned say that they cannot possibly use tampons.*

The reason for this is that suturing has been done too tightly, not allowing for the swelling that follows injury to tissue that is especially sensitive. If you have ever seen anyone with a wasp sting near the eye, you know how enormous the swelling is. Perineal tissue reacts in a similar way.

After an episiotomy it is impossible to have intercourse until everything has healed.* At three months more women who have had episiotomies have pain with attempted intercourse than do those who have had even severe tears. Those still in most pain are women who have had both an episiotomy and a tear.* A woman who cannot bear the thought of love-making because she is in pain often feels that it must be her own fault.

A small proportion of women, even after painstaking suturing, are left with a recto-vaginal fistula (a gap in the wall between the rectum and vagina) and pass faeces through the vagina. So they have another operation weeks or months later for the fistula to be repaired. The emotional as well as the physical effect of all this cannot be underestimated. They are left feeling mutilated, abused, and dirty. They may feel scalding anger or be deeply depressed.

After suturing some women suffer pain that continues for years. Sometimes this happens because the vagina has been stitched too tight, with the tissues stretched and aching. Sometimes nerves have been sliced through. Sometimes a large knob of scar tissue remains painful, and the woman feels as if she is sitting on thorns.

> "My husband is very patient and understanding but he thinks I should be better by now."

When she seeks professional help, she may be advised to lubricate the area that is painful, be told that the pain will pass eventually, be sent to a psychotherapist or marriage counsellor, or be offered surgery to cut out scar tissue and improve the "cosmetic" result.

When a woman gives birth at home or in a birth centre episiotomies are not done automatically. They are reserved for those situations in which a baby needs to be born quickly. Midwives have skills of "guarding" the perineum with a hand, enabling a woman to give birth slowly and gently, so that it is not over-stressed and there is less likelihood of a tear occuring.

Midwives also use hot compresses or warm water and often they use words, such as a fan opening wide, water flowing, or a flower spreading wide its petals, that suggest vivid visual images.* Many also use methods such as birth in water, which seems to help maintain the elasticity of a woman's perineum.

drugs and infection in hospitals

Two major inter-related problems in hospitals today are cross-infection and resistance to antibiotics. At home a woman can usually cope with bacteria in her own family. Moreover, since she is not exposed to obstetric intervention at home, damage to tissue, whether on the surface of her body or deep inside it, is unlikely to allow the introduction of harmful bacteria. The baby is resistant to many infections, both because of immunity built up through the placenta while inside the uterus and from maternal colostrum and breast milk after birth.

Pelvic, bladder, perineal and breast infections are normally treated with penicillin or related antibiotics. These drugs are highly effective if used when a woman has a Caesarean section (which brings with it an increased risk of contracting a pelvic infection as well as infection of the scar). But liberal use of penicillin produces resistant strains of disease.

Bacteria are clever and adapt rapidly to threat. "In 1941, 10,000 units of penicillin administered four times a day for four days cured patients of pneumococcal pneumonia", a specialist at Columbia University writes*. He says that today the patient could have 24 million units a day, and still die.

Hospitals started using antibiotics in the nineteen fifties. Today approximately one patient in every three is on antibiotics. We do not know how long it will be before there are so many genetically modified, penicillin-resistant strains that penicillin becomes useless. Some doctors are already claiming that we face a global epidemic.*

Newborn babies as patients

In hospital the moment that babies are born, and even before birth, they are treated as patients, and may be subjected to a range of painful practices which cause distress and interfere with their smooth adjustment to life. The babies find it hard to get the knack of breastfeeding and cry a great deal.

♦ In many hospitals the first assault on babies as they are born is to suction them, by passing a tube into the nose and mouth to extract any mucus that might be in the airways. This suctioning of the baby's nasal passages and throat is especially distressing for the baby when done roughly, using a catheter rather than a suction bulb.* It may result in cardiac arrhythmia and, if the catheter touches the larynx, is likely to cause laryngeal spasm. Occasionally the herpes virus or bacteria are transferred through the suction catheter to the baby from the midwife or doctor.* Even with babies who have already passed meconium (the first contents of the bowel) – a sign that they may be under stress – it is uncertain whether intubation does more good than harm.*

♦ In some hospitals another routine is to pass a tube down into the baby's stomach to clear any gastric secretions that may be there. This scouring of the baby's gastric tract is another assault. It leads to slowing of the heart-rate and spasm of the larynx, which can interfere with the baby's whole pattern of sucking and swallowing, so that feeding is made more difficult.*

♦ Some countries have a law that all newborn babies must receive prophylaxis against gonorrhoeal blindness. This is not the case in the UK. Silver nitrate drops are put in the baby's eyes. They are intensely irritating and cause babies to close their eyes, interfering with communication between the mother and her baby in the hour following birth, the time when the baby is most likely to be in a quiet, alert state.* In fact, erythromycin works better than silver nitrate* and is also effective against chlamydia, a sexually transmitted disease, which a baby can pick up from the mother's vagina.* Silver nitrate is not effective against chlamydia.

In hospital you may have little or no control over what is put in your baby's eyes because there are often hospital protocols which do not permit choice. At home this is something you decide together with your midwife.

tender, loving care?

In some hospitals large numbers of babies are moved to the special care nursery, if only for observation. In many countries babies are routinely separated from their mothers anyway, isolated in a small room with a large window where a nurse glances at them occasionally. I have seen this happening in Italy. They are in a large nursery under bright, fluorescent lights with dozens of other babies, as in the USA, or even in a good-sized cupboard which nurses use as a refuge where they can chat and smoke – something that I have observed in the USSR.

Apart from the emotional deprivation caused to the mother by taking her baby away from her immediately after the birth – the reward of all her work and striving – and the loneliness and confusion the baby may feel, this is bad practice. It can be dangerous. When babies are herded together in this way, the risk of cross-infection is high, and no one is likely to watch a newborn baby as unceasingly and with such acute observation as the baby's own mother.

"Every part of me seemed to fill with what I can only describe as "a loving ecstasy". This intense communication was never possible in hospital immediately after birth, as the babies were not beside me. But I wonder if there it could have taken place. It was something so special I think it needed exactly the right receptive conditions on both our parts for it to happen."

Babies are treated as if they are the property of the hospital rather than the mother, and as if trained professionals are the only people who could safely assess a baby's condition and give appropriate care. When the World Health Organization enquired in 24 European countries what the usual practices were, it was revealed that in 17 countries babies were automatically separated from their mothers for a period of time after birth.*

Bonding

Bonding is sometimes seen as something that must be "facilitated" or actively taught by staff, rather than as a process that cannot be rushed, that occurs in its own way and its own sweet time if a mother has her baby with her whenever she wants, for as long as she wants, and if she is in a supportive, friendly environment.

In some hospitals bonding theory has been incorporated into care in very destructive ways. Women say they feel they have to put on a performance and respond to their babies in the correct, loving style, because they are aware that they are under the scrutiny of staff checking to see if bonding is taking place.

"I knew they were watching me to see if we were bonding. But the birth had been such an ordeal I needed time. I couldn't be rushed. I felt I had to put on an act."

Being forced to take what amounts to an examination in motherhood within a few hours or even minutes of your baby's birth is not the best way of starting off a relationship. It interferes with the powerful emotions that may be sweeping through you, and is likely to make you self-conscious, self-questioning and inhibited. Most women overcome these obstacles. But it is hard on those who have had a stressful and difficult birth, and who may not be able to "come back into themselves" and feel secure enough to reach out to their babies. They need peace and quiet, and to be nurtured themselves, before they can nurture their babies.

A gentler alternative

Many hospitals now practice "gentle birth". Lights are dimmed for delivery, voices hushed, the baby is handled gently, and given to the mother immediately. She can cuddle her newborn against her bare skin under a special heater or a blanket which covers them both, and mother, father, and baby have uninterrupted time together for about an hour after the birth.

So far, so good. But what mothers often don't realize is that the baby may then be taken from them to another place for a paediatric examination. This is a brightly lit, noisy nursery – a very different environment from the close intimacy of that first postnatal hour.

At home, or in a birth centre, your baby remains with you and will never be taken away for any reason whatever, unless you wish it, and can stay with you in the same bed or close, right through the night, to be fed whenever she stirs. A mother watches her baby intently, fascinated by each tiny movement, and listens to the strange and sometimes quick, dancing patterns of breathing. What is happening is important in the development of the relationship between her and her baby. To interfere with or destroy that intimacy is to risk interrupting a vital psychological process that may reduce the woman's confidence in herself as a mother and interfere with the flow of communication between them.

"I want to spend time with the baby and my husband, talking about the whole experience and our feelings, without a time limit and without interference – in my own familiar surroundings."

39

safe home birth

Decisions about where to give birth should spring from realistic risk assessment and from your own values. Any woman who decides that birth without hospital is right for her, in a society that is hostile to freedom in childbirth, takes responsibility for weighing up risks. She also expresses the courage to resist autocracy, dogma and the power of the medical system. Her decision is based on deeply held values. Doctors, however, tend to see birth exclusively in terms of risk.

assessing risk

"You are high risk because you are 31 . . . it is your first baby and you have an untried pelvis . . . you had a miscarriage last year . . . you are in a high-risk ethnic group . . . you are single . . . this is your fifth baby . . . your last labour was induced and you had a forceps delivery . . . you have had a previous Caesarean section."

At the first antenatal visit the doctor may refer to a "risk score" to decide which category of care is appropriate for your pregnancy: this may be ordinary doctor/midwife, care under the direction of obstetricians, or highly specialized and intensive care from an expert team. You may have little choice in this. You are labelled high or low risk either on the basis of a score like this, or simply because of the doctor's clinical hunches. With some risk scores as many as nine out of ten women turn out to be classified as "high risk".

Attaching labels to pregnant women is damaging. A woman assigned to a high-risk category will probably have interventions that make birth more complicated, and women who are aware that they are "at risk" lose confidence and become anxious. If everyone around you expects things to go wrong, you begin to believe that they will – and they may well do so.

Often a woman is categorized as high or low risk without reference to her everyday life. Such things as poor housing, bad conditions in the workplace, little money for food, a violent partner, social isolation, unemployment, or family problems are social conditions which are at the roots of perinatal mortality (baby deaths) and morbidity (illness).

"People say, "How brave you are, having your baby at home!" I don't feel brave at all. I think they're the brave ones, to go into hospital, and risk all the things that are done to you there."

Assigning all black women to an "at risk" category is racially discriminatory. There are wide variations in the life-styles, economic circumstances, and the education of black women. Asian women who live in one area of London have no more baby deaths than the general population, whereas those in Bradford, in the north of England, are much more likely to suffer the death of a baby. It is not a matter of skin colour, but of socio-economic conditions.

Birth, like all other human activities, is never entirely risk-free. But most risk markers used are very poor predictors. Some doctors still believe, for example, that any woman with small feet must have a small pelvic outlet too, so may ask their patients what size shoes they wear, and those wearing size 3 are automatically categorized as high risk. Research shows that this is ridiculous.*

Women often feel trapped with care that is imposed on them, which is very different from what they would have chosen.

To make decisions about the care we want and the place of birth, we need full and accurate information about potential risks and then decide ourselves what to do. Some risk is acceptable. We may want to go on holiday, so we take a plane. We enjoy skiing or rock-climbing and accept the risk of a broken leg. The risks are worth it. If sailors worried about risk all the time, they would never go to sea.

We can also prepare to handle risks, taking sensible precautions against the most likely dangers, such as wearing a life-jacket on a sailing dinghy, or buckling on a safety belt in the car, and we can learn what to do if risks build up.

unravelling the statistics

It is often claimed that, because far fewer mothers and babies die than, say, 60 years ago when most women had their babies at home, hospital birth must be the cause of this. But the fact that two things happen at the same time does not mean that one causes the other.

Nor should we use statistics of home births from the past, or from Third World countries. Many things are different, including our health, access to contraceptives and abortion, and our socio-economic conditions. These have a profound effect on perinatal mortality. As the standard of living rises, fewer babies die at birth in every country, whether or not they are born in hospital.

Unplanned births outside hospital are often included in the statistics for home births, and this gives a completely wrong impression of the comparative risks of home and hospital births.

In 1980 the Social Services Committee of the British House of Commons recommended that more women should be delivered in large units and home birth "phased out further".* It based this policy on a graph showing that more babies died at home than in hospital. Hidden in those statistics was the fact that it was unplanned out-of-hospital births that accounted for the increase in deaths.*

Women who have unplanned out-of-hospital births may be delivering long before the baby is ready for life, or may be teenagers hiding a pregnancy and delivering somewhere, anywhere, where they hope their parents will not find out about the baby, or women delivering in panic on the way to hospital, or those who have had no antenatal care at all – the very poor, mentally confused, severely depressed, or drug addicted.

Home birth in different countries

All over the world Caesarean section rates are on the increase. In Britain they have more than doubled in a generation, and over 93,00 Caesareans are performed each year. Though it might be expected that Caesareans are replacing instrumental deliveries, this is not the case. Forceps and ventouse deliveries are also increasing. More and more women are having highly medicalised births.

At the same time women are expressing renewed interest in giving birth at home. In the Netherlands, where it is very safe to have a baby, it is a straightforward matter to arrange this, and one third of all women have home births. It remains an exceptional country. Yet even where women give birth under the most centralised and authoritarian medical systems, such as in Russia, women are wanting home births.

In Britain home births reached an all time low of less than 1 per cent in the 1980s, but are now on the increase. Five thousand women

Assessing risk

Q What equipment does the midwife carry?

A The midwife will have simple equipment such as a Pinard's stethoscope or a sonic aid, some pain-relieving drugs, and other drugs to make the uterus contract after the baby is born if you bleed heavily. She may have aromatherapy oils, transcutaneous electronic nerve stimulation apparatus (TENS) to help you cope with pain, or even a birth stool, or suggest that you get these things.

Q What happens if the baby has breathing problems?

A Babies are more likely to experience breathing difficulties if the mother has had pain-killing drugs in labour, especially pethidene. A woman may not have any drugs at all in a home birth. And if she does have pain-relieving drugs these are given in small doses. The midwife carries oxygen and simple resuscitation equipment in case it is needed.

Q I had a Caesarean last time, can I give birth at home this time?

A It will be more difficult to get a doctor or midwife to agree. There are additional risks in having a baby outside hospital, but there are also risks with the unnecessary and harmful interventions that can occur in hospitals. It may be that the previous Caesarean was the result of intervention, such as being induced, being stuck in bed, having an epidural, or fetal monitoring.

Q I am very overweight. Should I have a home birth?

A It helps to be within a normal weight range. But never go on a crash diet during pregnancy. This is bad for both you and your baby. Ask for help from a dietician.

Q I am an "older" first-time mum. Can I have a home birth?

A Though your doctor many not be encouraging, if you are healthy and have a normal pregnancy, there is no reason why you should not plan a home birth, though there is a higher chance of being transferred to hospital during the first stage of labour simply because it may take a long time.

Minimizing the risks

If you are going to have your baby at home, it makes sense to:

♦ Find a midwife you like. She should be skilled, confident, and relaxed in working in an out-of-hospital setting.

♦ Approach birth free from fear, self-assured and positive.

♦ Acquire the art of meeting contractions with relaxation, breathing and concentration, and learn about using different positions and movements.

♦ Have more than one birth attendant. Your caregivers need to work well together, and your midwife needs her own support. Think about having a doula, or birth companion. To find a doula see p.192–193

♦ Ensure you have access to a telephone, and a car as well, if possible.

♦ Consider hiring a birth pool. See p.192–193

a year have home births and the number is rising rapidly. In parts of the south west of England the proportion of home births is as high as 20% and many pregnant midwives themselves choose home births. The Department of Health forecasts that home births will be 7 per cent of all births by the year 2005. That amounts to more than 18,000 home births a year in England and Wales.

In the USA approximately 35,000 women a year give birth at home or in a free-standing birth centre. Many more would do so if there were the midwives to attend them, but midwives are few and far between. In Canada, following the legalisation of midwifery in some provinces, it is easier to get midwife care and midwives work both in hospitals and may attend home births.

In Western Australia professional caregivers working in hospitals are very disapproving of home births. As a result, women who seek home birth, especially those who have had previous unhappy hospital experiences, are reluctant to be transferred even when there is strong indication that it would be safer for them and their babies to switch to hospital. When they are admitted women are separated from their own midwives, who must wait outside, and they often encounter punitive attitudes. This conflict between philosophies, fought out by those who should be giving service to childbearing women, wherever they are, and whatever the circumstances, leads to confrontation, and to delays in treatment, with home birth midwives and hospital doctors trying to prove their point.

The Australian situation is very different from that in countries where there is an established home birth service. Wherever women have to fight to get home birth they may do so even when they are potentially at high risk, believing that doctors are not telling them the truth and will not respect their wishes if they go into hospital. In Western Australia, for example, as many as 43 per cent multiparous women who have home births had complications in previous births.* They were either ill-informed or were so scared of hospitals because of their previous experiences that they decided to take the risk. This is an indictment of a hospital system, not of the women who are abused by it.

Safety

It may be useful to look at the Netherlands, where 38 per cent of babies are still born at home. Women having babies at home there may be cared for by a midwife or a general practitioner, and in hospital by midwives or doctors. If you look at baby deaths both in

The care you give yourself in pregnancy is more important than anything offered by a clinic.

terms of where the birth took place and of who attended the birth it emerges that care given by a midwife at home is safer than care from midwives in hospital, and home birth with a midwife is safest of all.*

A meta-analysis, research based on the most reliable studies into planned home births in different countries, shows that home birth is a valid alternative if you are not at special risk of difficulties in childbirth, and also reveals that if you give birth at home you have fewer medical interventions. The research covered 24,092 home births, matched with births to low risk women who were planning birth in hospital.* Significantly fewer women who planned a home birth had their labours induced, received an episiotomy, or ended up with an operative vaginal delivery or Caesarean section. They were less likely to have a bad perineal tear, and their babies were in better condition at birth. The conclusion is: "Home birth is an acceptable alternative to hospital confinement for selected pregnant women, and leads to reduced medical interventions."

It can be difficult to have a normal birth in hospital. Research into 6,000 planned home births in England and Wales revealed that women were one hundred times more likely to have labour induced if they planned a hospital birth, only 7 per cent of women giving birth at home had their membranes artificially ruptured at or before 4 cms dilatation of the cervix, compared with 25 per cent of those in hospital, and 8 per cent received pethidine, compared with 30 per cent in hospital.* Four times as many hospital mothers had a prolonged labour, and twice as many had an operative vaginal birth or Caesarean section. Though few women actually haemorrhaged, twice as many women in hospital had heavy blood loss. At home women were more likely to have an intact perineum or, if they had a tear, only a first degree laceration, which is just a split in the skin, and does not damage muscle.

The babies did better at home too. Three times as many babies were recorded as having fetal distress in hospital. Twice as many had a low Apgar score (the examination that reveals if a newborn is lively) and more than twice as many needed oxygen.

For low risk mothers home birth is as safe, for both mother and baby, as hospital birth. In fact, it may be safer.

a closer look at risks

Smoking

If you smoke, the single most important thing you can do to reduce risk to yourself and your baby is to stop smoking before you get pregnant, or in the first half of the pregnancy, or, at least, cut it down below ten cigarettes a day. Many midwives in the USA and Canada will not accept home birth clients who smoke during pregnancy, because of the associated risks.

Nicotine constricts blood vessels so that the flow of blood through the placenta is slower, and this can lead to intra-uterine growth retardation (IUGR). Carbon monoxide and thiocynate in cigarette smoke also reduce the baby's growth. Smokers are more at risk of miscarriage, of having preterm babies, and of haemorrhage from the placenta. A woman who smokes and also drinks alcohol takes even greater risks.

Alcohol

In North America fetal alcohol syndrome is the most usual teratogenic cause (that is, damage caused while the baby is in the uterus) of mental handicap. This may occur when a woman drinks around eight glasses of wine or four pints of beer a day. You don't have to drink this much, however, to make it more likely that a baby will be born with low birth weight. There is some evidence that if you drink more than ten glasses of wine a week the baby does not grow so well in the uterus.*

Your weight

If you are very underweight or overweight, this may affect your pregnancy and labour too. If you are very underweight, there is a chance that the baby will not be well nourished. If you are very fat, you are more likely to have raised blood pressure and to develop pregnancy diabetes, both of which will lead to your being advised not to give birth at home.*

Being fat means that you are also more likely to develop a urinary infection or to have a blood clot during pregnancy. But if you are healthy, there is no added risk to the baby; healthy overweight women give birth to healthy babies.* The customary practice of being weighed regularly in pregnancy, and all the worry that results, is worse than useless.

Your blood pressure

It is natural for blood pressure to rise a little at the very end of pregnancy.* But, if your blood pressure is up and at the same time protein (albumen) appears in your urine, you have preeclampsia and, unless it is very mild, will usually be advised to have your baby in hospital, because the placenta may not be functioning well.

If your blood pressure is rising, look at ways in which you can cut down stress and take life easier. Pamper yourself and, if you possibly can, go to bed and ask other people to shop, cook, and clean. Listen to music, read, practise your relaxation, and get someone you love to massage you with a relaxing aromatherapy oil. If you already have children, this is very difficult to do unless there are other people close to you who can take over the children. You can always cuddle up with a toddler in bed, with picture books, television, and some new playthings, but two-year-olds are not the most restful little people to have around, and the therapy for your high blood pressure will have to be a compromise between care for yourself and the joys and responsibilities of mothering. But, however you work it out, getting more rest gives you the best chance of being healthy at the end of the pregnancy, and still being able to have your baby at home. If this is your first baby, remember that once the baby is born you will never have the opportunity to lie around luxuriously like this again, so enjoy it!

A breech baby

Three or four babies in every 100 are born bottom first.* Problems can arise because, although the baby's body may slip through easily, the birth of the head may be delayed, and this can result in oxygen deprivation.

In some countries Caesarean sections are performed for most breech births, on the grounds that it is better to be safe than sorry. In Sweden nine out of ten breech babies are Caesarean births. Compare this with Norway, where only four or five are caesareans. If you know that if you have your baby in hospital you are bound to have a Caesarean, you may feel that a home or birth-centre birth is an alternative, so long as you can arrange for skilled and experienced care. However, you may find that your caregivers are very reluctant to take on the extra risk of a breech birth. It is important that your midwife feels confident.

More than 30 per cent of breech babies are born like this because they are pre-term (not yet 37 weeks). It is only as a baby becomes heavier that it tips head-down.

Babies who are breech in late pregnancy often somersault and are head-down by the time labour starts. About 14 per cent are breech at 32 weeks,* and there is a three in five chance of them turning after that time, and still at 36 weeks a one in four chance,* though this is less likely if the baby's legs are extended, because legs splint the body, making it harder for the baby to roll over. Some babies even kick themselves round once labour has actually started, provided that they have enough space.

External version in late pregnancy is successful in 60 per cent of cases. It is a simple, safe alternative to Caesarean section.* Be sure to ask for this if your baby is breech and you plan a home birth.

A previous pre-term baby

If you have had a baby before who was born pre-term, there is an increased possibility that this will happen again, but you still have an 83 per cent chance of going to full term with this pregnancy.

Even if you have previously had two pre-term births, there is still a 72 per cent chance it will not happen with this pregnancy.*

A previous Caesarean

If you have had a previous Caesarean section, you will be advised by doctors to have your next baby and all other babies in hospital. Many obstetricians in North America do a repeat Caesarean even when the same problems do not recur in another labour. This is one reason why the Caesarean section rate has multiplied five times in the last 20 years.

British obstetricians adopt a different approach. They allow a "trial" of labour. This is really a trial of the scar, with everything ready for Caesarean section in case it splits. That means a hospital birth.

Rupture of the uterus occurs extremely rarely. In a series of 110,000 births following previous Caesarean section there were a total of 13 ruptures.*

Most of the papers in medical journals on which doctors base their policies warn against rupture following the old-fashioned "classical" Caesarean section, when the incision in the uterus is vertical. Nowadays most incisions are horizontal, in the lower segment of the uterus, just about at the level of the top of a bikini.

The risks of the scar rupturing are much reduced when a horizontal, lower-segment incision has been made and, even when the scar does not stand up to the strain, it does not pop open, but one edge unpeels slightly.

medical conditions

Sometimes pregnant women are told by doctors that, if they suffer from certain illnesses, such as diabetes, they must give birth in hospital. They can make a strong case for diabetic mothers because, with all that sugar in the blood, babies often grow very large. In the past babies of diabetic mothers often had breathing problems. But, now that there is good insulin control during pregnancy, fewer than 2 in 100 have breathing problems.*

If you have an illness that gets worse when you are under stress, however, home may be the best place for you if you feel more secure and confident there. With asthma, for example, there is no increased risk to the baby, and a good case for having a baby at home.* With multiple sclerosis, home may be the ideal place too.*

You are Rhesus negative

Your blood is tested for the Rhesus factor in early pregnancy. If you are Rhesus negative and the baby's father is Rhesus positive, you have further tests later in pregnancy to find out whether you are developing antibodies to a Rhesus positive baby. This is extremely unlikely to happen if it is your first baby and if you have not had a previous miscarriage, but the risk increases if anything is done that causes bleeding in pregnancy, such as chorionic villus sampling, amniocentesis, and fetoscopy.

Interventions during labour and at delivery can also cause leaking of the baby's blood into your own and result in sensitization in the next pregnancy. These include fixing a scalp clip to the baby's head to monitor the heart-rate, forceps delivery or Caesarean section, accidental tearing of the cord if it is pulled in an attempt to deliver the placenta, and manual removal of the placenta. So childbirth without unnecessary intervention is the safest course of action, which may mean that birth at home or in a birth centre is best.

The discovery of gamma-globulin in the 60s, and its regular use now when a Rhesus negative woman is likely to be bearing a Rhesus positive baby, has saved many lives. You have injections of

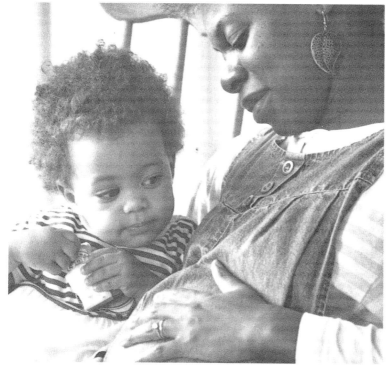

Each pregnancy is unique. A woman who has had a difficult one first time around may thoroughly enjoy her next pregnancy.

anti-D immunoglobulin during pregnancy, at the birth, or within five days of the birth of a Rhesus positive baby to avoid sensitization in the next pregnancy, and will be screened regularly during later pregnancies.

Fewer than one baby in 1,000 dies today from problems associated with Rhesus incompatibility. If you do not develop antibodies during pregnancy, your baby and you are not at increased risk. You should be able to choose the place where you would like to have your baby.

myths about home birth

"If you are an older mother you shouldn't have a home birth."

If you are having your first baby over the age of 35, or with some doctors even over 30, you are considered an "elderly primigravida", at greater risk of what obstetricians sometimes call "poor obstetric performance". Some even describe older mothers as "obstetrically senescent" or "geriatric".*

Nowadays women having their first baby in their thirties have not necessarily had a long history of fertility problems – something associated with increased risk – but have delayed motherhood because of their careers or until they felt ready to have a child. Their education and socio-economic conditions mean that they are in a low-risk group compared with, say, teenagers who become pregnant accidentally or because they want someone to love. The perinatal mortality rate for these older mothers is no higher than that for younger mothers.*

What is different is the amount of obstetric intervention that older mothers receive in hospital. In one London hospital women over 35 are more than twice as likely to have labour augmented with oxytocin (53 per cent compared with 20 per cent of under-35s), to have an episiotomy (74 per cent compared with 38 per cent), to be delivered by forceps (35 per cent compared with 25 per cent) or to have a Caesarean section (28 per cent compared with 13 per cent).* The high Caesarean rate may occur because more older mothers receive continuous electronic monitoring, and anxiety on the part of obstetricians may contribute to the aggressive management of labour. One way of avoiding this, a valid option if you have a healthy pregnancy, is to have your baby in a birth centre or at home.

"A long labour at home is dangerous."

It is tiring when the cervix dilates slowly but, unless other problems develop, this is not dangerous. Labours that last more than 48 hours in hospital often lead to forceps delivery, vacuum extraction, or Caesarean section, which may themselves introduce risk. At home you can have a more relaxed attitude to time. There is no relation between long labour (over 24 hours) and mental handicap in babies.*

Cephalo-pelvic disproportion (CPD.), where the baby's head is too big to pass through the mother's pelvis, is often misdiagnosed simply because labour is long. When a woman is in labour in her own home and it becomes obvious that the baby is having difficulty passing through her pelvis it is sensible to transfer to hospital. This is not a sudden emergency. It is a decision that can be made following discussion with your midwife when it is clear that no progress is being made.

A doctor having her first baby:
"Midwives carry oxygen to give a baby if necessary, but the doctors I saw didn't realize that. I want a home birth because I am anxious to avoid my delivery becoming as medicalized as those I witnessed during my training."

"If the baby has breathing problems nothing can be done."

Babies are most likely to have breathing difficulties when their mothers have had pain-killing drugs in labour, including pethidine, sedatives, tranquillizers, and epidural anaesthesia. A woman having a baby at home often has no drugs at all during her labour or, if she chooses to have them, has only a very small dose. Simple ways of resuscitating a baby – clearing the airways, giving oxygen and massage – can be used at home.

"You may haemorrhage."

Postpartum haemorrhage (heavy bleeding) is most likely to occur when there has been obstetric intervention in birth or attempts have been made to pull the placenta out before it has completely separated from the uterine wall. If there is bleeding, syntometrine (artifical oxytocin) can be given by injection to make the uterus contract firmly, and it is simple to do this at home.

The baby's safety

Whenever a woman decides to have a home birth, there are people who suggest that either the baby might die from neglect because it is not born in a hospital setting, or that it might be mentally damaged from lack of oxygen. In England and Wales perinatal mortality rate for planned home births is very low indeed – 3 to 4 per 1,000 compared with 8 per 1,000 births as a whole.

Moreover, two of these three or four deaths are unavoidable wherever the baby is born, because the baby is extremely pre-term or suffers a congenital handicap that is incompatible with life. All that birth in a high-tech hospital might do is delay death by a few days or weeks.

Ninety-two per cent of all mental handicap in babies occurs before labour, either as the result of congenital malformation (around 63 per cent) or of events and processes that occurred during pregnancy, such as intra-uterine growth retardation (8 per cent), infections such as rubella (6 per cent), or accidents such as lead poisoning. The damage occurred long before labour started.*

In a hospital with an intensive care unit a severely handicapped baby is taken immediately for all life-saving procedures that are available to be employed. Being in hospital may make the difference between death and survival with a major handicap. Some women choose home birth because they would not want vigorous and extraordinary methods to be used to save the life of a damaged baby. Others choose hospital because they want the baby to have every chance of life, however severe the handicap.

> "Working in an intensive care unit, I see many babies being kept alive who I think should have been allowed to die in peace. That's one reason why I've decided on a home birth."

taking control

It is an enormous responsibility to bring a baby into the world, and it starts long before the baby is in your arms. There are doctors who accuse women having home birth of "child abuse", and who would even like to prosecute them. They see it as a choice only a selfish woman would make, and see themselves as the saviours of babies, rescuing them from their egotistical, hysterical mothers. Yet your informed decision to give birth at home or in a birth centre can be one way to accept deep personal responsibility for your baby.

Charlotte's home birth

Charlotte is a schoolteacher, and this is her third baby.

She had a show, but for the following 48 hours had contractions only when she moved around.

To get labour going she and her birth companion, Janet, went for a long walk in nearby woods the next afternoon. But regular contractions, five minutes apart, did not start till late evening. She called her midwife at 11 p.m., who examined her and said, "You're not at all dilated." So she went to bed. At 4.30 a.m. powerful contractions woke her. "But because someone in authority had told me I was not dilating, I couldn't take them seriously. It was only at 7.15 a.m., when I tried to read the children their third morning story, that I thought, "I must do something about this!" Suddenly it was as if the labour jumped two gears. She crouched on the floor, feeling pulled down by gravity, and swayed, rocked, and groaned. "I have never felt anything so strong." The two midwives turned up at 8.30 a.m. By then she was kneeling with her arms on the bed. One of them examined her: "I had a vision of jumping out of the window if I was not dilating." But she was fully dilated. "I knew exactly what I was doing. I hardly had to push at all. It wasn't painful, and the baby slipped out in a calm, very controlled way at 8.40 a.m. It was wonderful!"

"I couldn't believe that here was a beautiful, healthy baby. I was completely bowled over! I laughed. There was a huge welling up of happiness. I feel I have been celebrating ever since – a bubbly feeling, like the fizz in champagne."

"Janet made me feel cherished. Her support during labour was important because I knew that she would not collude with doctors. Here was an ally. If I couldn't articulate what I wanted, she could articulate for me. She cherished me afterwards, too. She "happened to be passing – with a meal" and asked, "Can I share it with you?" I spent a week surrounded by women to whom I was close. They camped out here, and we had picnics."

"Imogen is Janet's baby as well as mine. We were on the same wavelength. When you share birth with another woman, you know that she understands with a great deal more clarity than a man what you are feeling or thinking. There was something about being surrounded by women, all giving loving support, that was very comforting. It felt secure, warm, and very strong. It was something that we all did together."

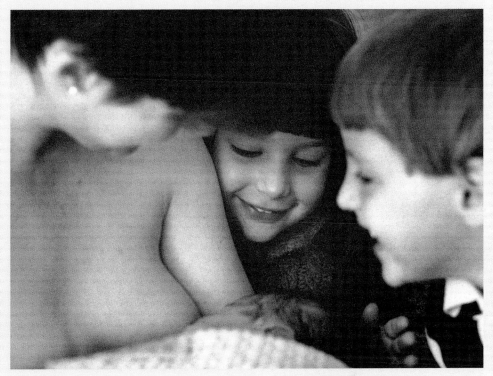

"It made the birth special to have the children there so quickly after, and to be able to share their wonder. I needed them. I couldn't have borne to be parted from them. And it was wonderful to sleep afterwards in a big bed with all my children."

Louise is five and William three-and-a-half. They came in immediately after the baby slipped out, and were fascinated by her. Louise went to school next day "just shining, from top to toe".

Charlotte freshened up in a warm bath, with the baby nestled close to her.

arranging a birth without hospital

Depending on where you live, you may have the choice between giving birth in a birth centre run by midwives, linked with or completely separate from a hospital, a small GP unit, or at home. It is worth exploring your options.

the birth centre: home from home?

A birth centre, at least ideally, provides exclusively low-technology care, there is a homely and relaxed atmosphere, and you return home a matter of hours after giving birth if you wish. In the United States, where the first one was established in New York in 1975, birth centres have mushroomed. Caregivers are for the most part nurse-midwives, direct-entry midwives, or nurses working with an obstetrician.

A birth centre may be free-standing, in hospital grounds, or inside a hospital building. The important thing about it is that it should have a distinct atmosphere of its own and its special staff. The policy of the Family Health Program Birth Center in Salt Lake City, for example, is "to provide safe maternity care to low-risk families, in a homelike, out-of-hospital setting," and achieve "parental satis-faction through a highly educational, personalized form of care, which encourages intrafamily contact and participation in the management . . . of childbearing. Childbirth is a peak life experience and is viewed as a healthy process. Confidence in the physiologic function of the body to cope with childbirth is promoted in all aspects of care." Health care providers are educators and resource people to enable women to take responsibility for their own health.

Some hospitals have introduced birth rooms with paintings on the walls, flowered wallpaper, hanging plants and rocking chairs, but there is no special philosophy of care that arises from a holistic approach to childbirth, and as much obstetric intervention is likely to take place in these rooms as in the more clinical-looking rooms along the corridor.

How is a birth centre different from a hospital?

In a birth centre worthy of the name, there is:

♦ No induction.

♦ No augmentation of labour with oxytocin.

♦ No electronic fetal monitoring except for Doppler ultrasound – the sonic aid.

♦ No drugs for pain relief except local analgesia to suture tears in the perineum.

♦ Very few episiotomies.

♦ No operative deliveries.

♦ In many birth centres the only equipment is oxygen, and catheters for clearing a baby's airways when they are blocked.

In the Garden of Life Birth Center in Dearborn, Michigan, where the focus is on cultural sensitivity to the needs of the Muslim, Italian, Hispanic, Polish and Anglo parents using the centre, the sole machinery is a coffee-maker. Staff wear ordinary clothing, not uniforms. Women can move around in labour and adopt any position they like for birth. Childbirth education is an integral part of the programme, and other members of the family can be present at the birth. The bed is king-sized, low, and comfortable, so that mother, father, and new baby can cuddle together.

"I saw my baby's head crowning and she was placed on my tummy. No tubes were forced down her throat. She was born amid laughter and joy, shared by all. Our second child is almost due and will be born in the same peaceful, gentle atmosphere of Boothville."

Midwives and nurses working independently in birth centres and small clinics, even in countries where midwifery is already a strong profession, as in Sweden, find a satisfying new role and exciting relationship with the families they are helping. In a birth centre in Stockholm, for example, it is a midwife, not a doctor, who makes the decision as to whether labour is deviating from the normal and who then refers a woman to obstetric care in the same building. In this birth centre such a referral happens with one woman in ten during pregnancy. In the early days a further 30 per cent of women were moved during labour, often for oxytocin stimulation of the uterus because their waters had broken and there were no contractions following membrane rupture, or labour was slow, but as midwives became more confident this very high percentage of transfers was halved in the first six months. In most American birth centres between 7 and 16 per cent of women are switched to regular obstetric care because they require drugs for pain relief, have slow labours, or there is failure to progress. You will need to bear this in mind if you decide you would like to give birth in a birth centre.

> "I enjoyed being looked after as a Special Mum, as everyone was treated there, and I treasure the warmth and fun that was shared with those midwives and doctors."

In England, the Edgware Birth Centre where 387 women gave birth over a two year period, only 6 had an episiotomy. That is a rate of 1.5 per cent compared with a rate of 11 per cent for women who had normal births in local hospitals. Half of the birth centre mothers gave birth in a pool.*

Why choose a birth centre?

In Britain, birth centres – both within the National Health Service and privately run, but often selling their service to NHS trusts – are now part of a rapidly developing movement aimed at woman-centred care. They fill the gap that resulted from the closing down of many small maternity units served by midwives and G.P.s and the difficulty that women experience in getting home births. All over the country these small birth units have been closed on the grounds that they are uneconomical and that it is safer for all births to be concentrated in large regional hospitals. The evidence for the increased safety of low risk mothers in large hospitals is unconvincing, and these cottage-hospital type birth units were held in great affection in their communities, but they were shut down all the same. Their destruction has left a huge gap. Women may have to travel great distances to hospital, are less likely to be able to get to know the midwives who attend them in childbirth, and the intimacy and friendliness of care is often lost in the large institutions which replaced them.

> 'It is a relaxed, caring, warm and friendly environment where you count as a person and not a number on a conveyor belt'.

Now birth centres are eagerly sought by women who dislike the impersonality of hospital, want to have people around them whom they know, to retain control over what happens to them,

A birth centre

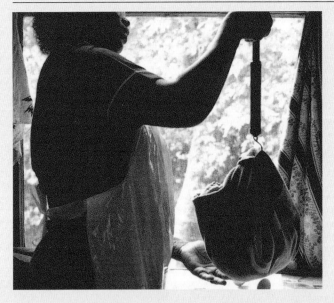

have a private room, with soft lighting, comfortable furniture, and equipment that enables you to be upright and to move around during labour. No shining instruments are in evidence, (though there may be some behind the curtain). You can bring things you would like to have and wear your clothes.

Q A **What is antenatal care like?**

Antenatal care is from midwives who give one-to-one care, discuss with you the emotional aspects of the birth experience, and do not limit care to doing tests and recording results. In some birth centres you are also shown how to check your own urine and blood pressure at home.

Q A **Can anyone use a birth centre?**

Birth centres are for low-risk women. If you are expecting twins, have pre-eclampsia or diabetes, or develop pregnancy problems, you will be excluded from giving birth there. Ask what the transfer rate is. A transfer rate in labour of 7 to 12 per cent is reasonable.

Q A **Are all birth centres run along the same lines?**

No. A set of rooms in a hospital decorated to look attractive, and that is not run by midwives, is a birth centre in name only.

Q A **Are birth centres safe?**

Birth centres have proved themselves safe, and in most, few invasive, uncomfortable, restrictive procedures are used. In the United States a study of 11,814 women admitted to 84 freestanding birth centres revealed that the perinatal mortality rate was as low as 1.3 per 1,000 births* compared with 8 per 1,000 for all hospital births.

Q A **What sort of atmosphere can I expect?**

The atmosphere is relaxing and non-clinical, and there is little or no intervention. You

Q A **And postnatal care?**

Your baby is able to stay with you through the 24 hours. So can your partner. You are given strong support for breastfeeding. You and your partner can be private – even lock the door, and your other children and family members are welcomed.

and labour without drugs or interventions. The Edgware Birth Centre, in London, for example, which is within the NHS, is booked solid and cannot keep up with demand.

It is not just pregnant women who may prefer birth in a small midwife-run centre. Midwives, lacking job satisfaction in large hierarchical, bureaucratic systems in which their skills are downgraded, look to these birth centres as places where they can give the kind of care which was the reason why they entered the profession. For some they hold the promise of a rebirth of midwifery.

In a good birth centre you can expect architecture on a human scale and attractive interior design, with such things as comfortable furniture, photographs of the midwives with their names on the notice board, and many photographs of mothers with their new babies, pictures, sculptures, mobiles, and other representations of birth and womb-ripeness. Rooms are often carpeted, lighting can be dimmed, there are curtains at the windows, beanbags and relaxation chairs, maybe a patchwork quilt, and a wooden crib or muslin-hung cot. You have your own bathroom with a large bath tub, perhaps a jacuzzi, and a powerful shower for back massage. There may be a birth pool in which you can labour and give birth if you wish.

The kitchen is often located centrally in the building and is a gathering-place for expectant parents, midwives, and new parents as they talk over cups of tea. In the Stockholm Birth Centre parents have their own fridge and make meals when they want them. No one serves up meals at set times. The father or mother, or perhaps a grandparent, makes a snack whenever they wish. In a very different birth centre in El Paso, Texas, the kitchen is also the heart of the centre – but, in contrast to the style of the modern white-wood Swedish kitchen with its bundles of dried rosebuds, this is a Mexican kitchen, familiar and comforting for the mothers who walk across the border in labour to give birth in the United States, and hope that in this way their babies may become American citizens. Instead of Swedish cheese and shortbread cookies, you sniff the odours of Mexican dishes based on black beans and peppers.

Choosing a good birth centre

There are phoney birth centres. As health care entrepreneurs and hospital administrators have caught on to the birth centre as a major marketing opportunity, a venture that could make their hospital more competitive with others, in the USA the original concept has been diluted. Those who own a birth centre – business people, doctors, a health authority, hospital, or whatever – control how it is run and everything that happens in it. If a birth centre is not run by the midwives who work in it, be particularly careful about examining the pros and cons. In US birth centres as a whole, 15 per cent of women have intravenous infusions, though only 8 per cent have episiotomies. The typical Californian centre is physician-owned in a commercial building, with a couple of birth rooms, and births are attended by the obstetricians. Californian physician-owned insurance companies will not usually provide malpractice cover for birth centres unless they are on hospital grounds, and only obstetricians can do deliveries. Malpractice insurance is too high for most family practitioners to risk working in a birth centre, and nurse-midwives have great difficulty in obtaining insurance cover to work in birth centres unless they are supervised by an obstetrician.

> "It's run by a cosmetic surgeon, with an obstetrician on call. He has an office downstairs where he does the cosmetic surgery."

In the United States, non-profit institutions staffed by nurse-midwives or registered midwives with back-up from a sympathetic obstetrician are giving way to hundreds of centres which are run for profit, and, as in Australia, hospitals offer birth rooms as a cosmetic exercise to attract more customers. Yet the non-profit birth centres that can still be found often provide the most value for money: offering more childbirth education, more prenatal care, more classes for siblings, and more home visits after the birth.

> "I was told that every first-time mother had Demerol (pethidine). It wasn't a question of whether she thought she needed it."

Along with the increase in physician-operated centres, some American obstetricians have equipped their offices to do out-of-hospital births, both in response to consumer demand and to make a fast buck. Procedures may include paracervical blocks (pain-killing injections around the cervix), electronic fetal monitoring, ultrasound, induction and augmentation of labour, vacuum extraction, forceps, and even, in at least one birth centre, Caesarean section.

As obstetricians take over the birth centre movement, they also transfer their concept of birth as a medical event, and with it increasing dependence on technology.

Questions to ask

When enquiring about a particular birth centre, you may want to ask these questions:

♦ What is your transfer rate during pregnancy? (This will enable you to estimate what your chances are of actually having your baby in the birth centre.)

♦ What is your transfer rate during labour? (A rate of between 7 and 12 per cent is reasonable.)

♦ Do you ever induce labour with oxytocin and/or amniotomy?

♦ Is electronic fetal monitoring used? (Doppler ultrasound, in the form of a hand-held sonic aid, for intermittent monitoring is acceptable. Scalp clips and abdominal belts are not.)

"There is a time-limit on labour, and then they shove you in a hospital. This hospital has a 30 per cent Caesarean section rate."

♦ Is intravenous glucose given?

♦ Are pain-relieving drugs used?

♦ Do you offer epidural anaesthesia?

♦ Is labour ever augmented with oxytocin?

♦ Is there a time limit on the second stage?

♦ What percentage of women have episiotomies? (It should be less than 10 per cent.)

♦ Do you ever do forceps delivery or vacuum extraction?

The answers to these questions may make you want to ask more. If any of these procedures are used, it will help to know if they are employed more or less routinely or rarely, so you may wish to ask for percentages of different interventions in the previous year.

Other questions concern your freedom to do whatever you feel like doing at the time:

♦ Can I walk around during labour?

♦ Can I give birth on the floor if I wish?

♦ Do women ever give birth standing up?

♦ How do you help a woman who is having a backache labour?

♦ Can I get in the bath or shower during labour?

♦ What do you do when dilatation is slow?

♦ Is it possible for my other children to be present?

♦ May I eat and drink during labour if I want to?

♦ Will there be a midwife with me all the time throughout the late first stage?

♦ Can I use a birth pool?

The answers will give you an idea of the quality of care, but your spontaneous feelings are also a good guide. Your intuitive reactions about whether this is the place in which you would like to give birth are important. You need to feel relaxed, confident, secure, and among friends.

In New York, outcomes for low-risk mothers booked at the Maternity Center's Childbearing Center were compared with those for low-risk mothers at a large teaching hospital, Mount Sinai.* Women in hospital were more likely to have labour induced, and augmentation of labour occurred six times as frequently. Amniotomy more than two hours before the birth was more common, electronic fetal monitoring was used five times as often, four times as many women laboured with intravenous drips set up, more than double the number had drugs for pain relief, and there were eleven times as many epidurals. Women in the birth center had noticeably longer second stages: over 80 per cent had second stages lasting more than two hours, compared with fewer than 19 per cent in the hospital. The incidence of thick meconium staining was three times greater for women in the hospital. (When some of the contents of the baby's bowel appear like this during labour, it can be a sign that the baby is over-stressed.) Women in the birth center were four times as likely to have an intact perineum: that is, no tear and no episiotomy. Judging by live, healthy babies, birth was just as safe in the Childbearing Center as at this prestigious hospital, but with far less intervention and in a pleasanter environment.

"Everything was warm, friendly, and fuss-free. My husband was tired after a long flight, and as I was walking about and leaning on Sue, my midwife, when I had a contraction, and was in and out of the bath, she tucked him up in the bed for a snooze whilst we got on with it. Then, when contractions were coming every two minutes, she woke him up with a cup of tea so that he didn't miss anything. She showed him how to rub my back and we made a great team!"

In hospitals, even those advocating "family-centred" care, intervention rates are much higher. Research in Australian hospitals reveals that those with flexible policies aiming for sensitivity to parents' wishes still have high rates of induction of labour, oxytocin use, and operative deliveries.*

In birth centres or birth rooms that are an integral part of a hospital the orientation towards treating patients as high-risk and using all techniques available spills over to low-risk women across the corridor. This takes place even though the benefits are marginal or non-existent and the interventions are sometimes harmful. In a

Canadian hospital, for example, as many as 63 per cent of first-time mothers and 19 per cent of those who had already had babies were transferred from the birth room to the conventional hospital setting.* Clearly, if you are choosing a birth centre linked to a hospital, it is essential that it has its own staff and that they are confident and skilled enough to give continuing, low-technology care.

GP units – small is beautiful?

Small general practitioner units are often homely and welcoming. Women like them because they already know the midwives and doctor, mothers and babies are kept together after the birth as a matter of course, and they are near home.

It is usually not possible to have an epidural or Caesarean section in a small unit like this, and a baby who needs special care must be moved to a larger hospital where there are intensive care facilities available. The emphasis is usually on as little intervention as possible during birth and on a close, supportive relationship between the midwife and her client.

> "The doctor tried to persuade me to go into the GP unit. He said it was "homely" and I could do just what I wanted there. But there's a vast difference between someone else's place being "homely" and my own home."

Isolated GP units have a good safety record. In New Zealand, for example, babies of normal birth weight are more likely to die in large, high-tech hospitals than in small maternity units.*

Choosing a GP unit

If you are considering a GP unit, visit it first and ask the same questions that you might ask of a birth centre (see page 65), including the rate of transfer. You will probably have a one-to-one relationship with the midwife because she is attached to your GP's practice, and will be able to ask her how she avoids episiotomies, what she recommends if a woman has a slow, backache labour, how she feels about water birth, and so on. With a good midwife this type of dialogue is a vital part of the relationship between you. Midwives create the flavour of a GP unit. In some areas they are attached to the GP unit rather than to GP practices, so you may not meet them unless you go to the unit.

Protocols for GP units are usually strict. You won't find high-tech gadgets sneaked in or interventionist obstetric techniques employed, although you may find that an amniotomy is done. It is likely that you will find midwives who are keen for you to walk about during labour or soak in a bath, and who know how to help you have a physiological rather than a managed birth.

You may have the option of a small maternity unit that is staffed and run by midwives, although few such clinics exist. They are very similar to those GP units that are separate from large hospitals, and the atmosphere is warm, friendly and relaxed. There is usually a good system of obstetric back-up combined with personal care from midwives whom you get to know before the birth.

Unfortunately, as we have seen, in most industrialized countries in Europe, North America, and Australia governments are closing down small hospitals and outlying GP units – in spite of a great deal of protest from consumers – on the grounds of safety, "rationalization", and economics. They are concentrating care instead in large regional centres that have high-tech facilities, great gleaming edifices of steel and glass. With regionalization of care, women then have to travel for long distances to antenatal clinics and once they have started labour. Moreover, care in these hospitals is focused on pathology, and tends to be less flexible and more impersonal than in small hospitals. There is often severe overcrowding in the antenatal clinics, with long waiting times, and women are herded through the clinics like cattle. Authoritarian attitudes set administrative convenience before the needs of the women for whom the service is supposed to exist.*

> There is a genuine friendship with a doctor who shares your conviction that home is the best place, and who supports you.

Many GP units have, at least potentially, the qualities of a good birth centre and offer a similar relaxed kind of care. Without the chance of either of these options, women are forced into standard hospital care, with its high intervention rates, unless they decide on home birth.

If you are considered sufficiently low-risk to be allowed to give birth in any of these small maternity units, however, you might also think about the option of home birth. If it is a sensible choice to give birth in a unit like this, it is equally safe, or even safer, to give birth at home.

One of the strongest arguments against having your baby anywhere else is that once a woman is in an institution interventions can take place that no midwife or doctor would be likely to attempt at home. Even in small maternity units there is a

GP Units

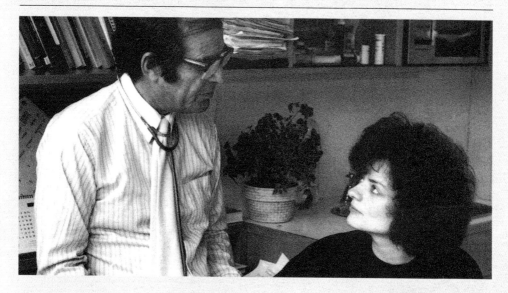

Q What is a GP unit?

A General practitioner units, sometimes isolated, such as exist in the UK and other European countries, and in Australia and New Zealand, grew out of cottage hospitals serving the community. They are really midwifery units. There are 55 freestanding midwifery units like this in England. They cater for low-risk women only.

Q Will I be able to have an active birth?

A Some of these small hospitals are quite old-fashioned, but many have kept the best of the old and incorporated active childbirth and gentle birth into their practice.

Q Will my GP look after me?

A No. Although they are called "GP beds", most care is by midwives. The GP may not even turn up for the birth.

Q Who can use a GP unit?

A They are for women who are expected to have normal births. The transfer rate to hospital because of unexpected complications is anything from 7 per cent to 30 per cent. It is worth asking what the transfer rate is.

Points to consider

- Is there a GP unit sufficiently close to my home?
- If I need to be transferred to hospital during the labour how far will I have to travel, and what kind of care can I expect from that hospital?
- Will I be able to choose the type of birth I want for myself and my baby and will I be free to make my own decisions?
- Will I have a chance to get to know my carers during pregnancy and discuss my choices for the birth before I go into labour?

risk that physiological labour is turned into managed labour just because you are in a place where medical hardware may be available, and where professionals make decisions without consulting you.

at home

The essential difference between giving birth at home and giving birth in even the most peaceful, pleasant birth room in an institution is the knowledge that home is your space, the place that you control, and where other people come as guests.

If you have decided that you will feel more secure, more confident, and more relaxed giving birth at home, the first step is to find out what is available in your area. In Britain you do not require a doctor's consent to have a home birth. You can make arrangements directly with a midwife. But, unless you live in a place where there are keen home birth midwives, arranging a home birth may not be easy.

"I went to my doctor expecting opposition and he said, "What a good idea!""

The first challenge may be to obtain information about who can help if your doctor refuses a home birth. One of the organizations listed on page 192–3 will be able to put you in touch with a group in your area. Working your way past other people's non-comprehension, criticism, and their sometimes punitive responses, may be rather like finding your way through a baffling maze. But it can also be exciting!

Talking to your doctor

Do not attempt to broach the subject when you are flat on your back with your legs in the air. Make certain that you are sitting face to face with the doctor. Settle back comfortably in the chair, avoid fiddling nervously with your clothes, hands, or bag, and look the doctor straight in the eye.

""You do realize", he said, "that home birth is child abuse? We've got a perfectly good hospital here offering family-centred care." "

Rehearse what you are going to say beforehand with someone sympathetic. It helps to have someone who knows what doctors may say in these situations. Remember that most doctors are frightened of home births because they have no experience of them. You don't have to go into lengthy explanations or make a speech, to defend or excuse yourself, to quote statistics, or to placate the doctor. Refuse to be drawn into arguments. All you need do is say clearly and firmly that you want a home birth, and, if you wish, give a simple explanation of why. You may have to repeat it over and over again, a technique sometimes known as "the cracked record". Afterwards discuss with the other person how you each felt at different stages of the conversation, and at the end of it.

"None of the local GPs was prepared to take me on, and we were summoned to see the chief obstetrician of the area, who underlined that a home birth was out of the question. We politely said that we should have been grateful for expert assistance at the delivery but, since this was not forthcoming, we preferred to take our chances at home. Several weeks later, out of the blue, a letter arrived informing us that three midwives had been assigned to us."

If you find this difficult, you can rehearse the interview by yourself, sitting in front of a mirror. Talk as if to the doctor, smiling and saying: "I should like a home birth." Then pause and listen attentively, imagining your doctor's reply. Then repeat your statement. Try this ten times. How did you sound . . . and look? Were you inclined to shout or whisper? Did you cross your arms so that you looked on the defensive? It is not only what you say, but how you say it, that is important. Your tone of voice can convey confidence or invite conflict or bullying. Practise saying, "I've decided that I want a home birth," in as many different ways as possible and settle for the tone and low pitch that makes you sound pleasantly assertive and friendly.

Once you get approval in principle, most doctors will want to know that you will agree to be transferred to hospital if there are signs that the baby is over-stressed. You can make it clear that you agree to this, provided that everything is explained to you and you don't feel that any decisions are being taken over your head. You may want to say that there are obviously situations in which this would be your choice too, but that you would not want to transfer to hospital just because labour was long and drawn-out. Be sure to keep copies of all correspondence concerning your request for a home birth.

For a woman who is disabled, home may be the best place because it is familiar, and she can feel free in a setting that she knows well and which is adapted to her needs. A woman with polyarthritis says, "A lot of disabled women are told, "You're disabled, so of course you go into hospital."

"What is important is the attitude you have to authority. To have a home birth, you have to be willing to question and to challenge authority."

You don't get any choice at all. But I'm assertive – when you've been in a wheelchair for two years, you know how to get your own way." She was firm that she wanted a home birth and a birth pool,

Being in your own surroundings allows you to feel comfortable and adopt whatever positions are best for you.

and found this the ideal solution. "Water encourages you to relax when you're disabled, and you're much freer in water. I just floated, with my boyfriend in the pool supporting me from behind. When we needed the midwives, they were there. When we wanted to be alone, we could be alone." She gave birth to a baby who rotated from the posterior position just before delivery, she had an intact perineum, and her baby was vigorously healthy and alert from the moment of birth.

"When you have a home birth, you don't have to go to someone else's place. It's your place. That makes all the difference."

Being assertive

If your doctor proposes a "compromise" solution — that you go into hospital for a short time and return home after a few hours, or are booked for a birth room, or suggests that care is modified to meet your special requests about not having drugs, or that electronic fetal monitoring will be used for only 20 minutes or so after you are admitted, and then you will be free to move around — and if you are not happy with that proposed compromise, say so and openly restate what you want.

On the other hand you may not want to say yes or no on the spot, and you can take time to think about it, discuss it with your partner, and then write to the doctor if you say, "I'd like a few days to consider that," "We need to talk this through," or "I'll think hard about that and let you know my decision next week." Do not be steam-rollered into an agreement that you may regret later.

Having said this, you do not have to put on a perfect performance. You have a right to be emotional, to get angry, to weep, to make mistakes, to be illogical, and even, if that is how it turns out, to be unassertive!

You are entitled to your own ideas about how you would like your birth to be. You are not on trial. You want the best for you and your baby. Whatever advice you are given, whatever the strength of other people's feelings, you have the right and responsibility to come to your own informed decision about where you have your baby.

What if my Doctor says "no" to a home birth?

If your GP is not happy with your decision, you can change your doctor, or be cared for by a midwife, perhaps with obstetric back-up directly from the hospital. You also have the right to decline medical intervention of any kind. The introduction of the provisions of the European Convention on Human Rights in 1988 * makes consent a matter of human rights and in the words of a Professor of Medical Law "respect of bodily integrity and privacy are values that are central to any theory of consent".*

Handling stress and keeping a cool head

It is sometimes stated that home birth is safe in the Netherlands because of careful selection. This is true. But it is selection of high-risk women for hospital, rather than selection for home birth. There birth is treated as normal process that can take place at home unless there are special reason why a woman is advised to go to hospital. In other countries selection is made for home birth and it is taken for granted that birth takes place in hospital unless a woman shows no deviation from a medically agreed and often rigidly defined "normal" down to the last detail.

Any woman wanting a home birth has to pass serial examinations to prove herself worthy of it. The testing is itself highly stressful. It may contribute to raised blood pressure and stress related illnesses, and increases her anxiety. It is difficult for even the most confident woman to take these examinations in her stride. So it is important to have strong support from someone close, a confiding friend with whom you can share your anxieties, to develop assertiveness skills in dealing with medical encounters, and obtain the knowledge on which you can make informed choices between alternatives from a birth organisation, midwifery and medical journals, books and the Web. You will find a list of organisations on page 193. Skills in handling stress include meditation, relaxation, rhythmic, controlled breathing, yoga, energetic physical activity, and creative work – anything that helps you feel in control of your own life and positive about your pregnancy.

How to handle stress

♦ Loving support from someone close who builds your confidence.
♦ A friend in whom you can confide your worries, and who is not judgemental.
♦ Relaxation and massage with aromatherapy oils.
♦ Meditation and positive fantasies about birth.
♦ Yoga. You may find a special class for pregnancy.
♦ Rhythmic breathing, not as an exercise, but at any time when you feel under stress.
♦ Physical activity: walking, swimming, gardening, cycling.
♦ Make things: any creative activity is good. Try making pictures, pots, tending the garden, baking, or making beautiful things for your baby.
♦ Assertiveness skills in difficult relationships. Ask your antenatal teacher for guidance, and perhaps help with role play.
♦ Accurate evidence-based information: read evidence-based books and papers. If you have access to the internet, visit useful sites and get as much information as you can (see page 193).

Organising a home birth

Q **What should I do once I have decided on a home birth?**
A
Visit your GP or go straight to a community midwife attached to a GP practice and say that you want a home birth.

Q **What if I am not on a GP's list?**
A
Contact a home birth support group, as the situation varies in different parts of the country (see page193).

Q **What if my GP refuses me a home birth?**
A
If you come to the decision that you want to give birth at home this is your right wherever you are in the UK. However, you may find that your GP is not willing to support your decision. The Royal College of General Practitioners advises that a GP should then refer you to another GP who does support home births.

Q **Who else can I turn to for help?**
A
You do not need a GP to have a home birth. Contact the Director of Midwifery saying that you intend to have a home birth and request a midwife. Again, a home birth support group can advise you what to do.

Q **How can I arrange antenatal care?**
A
Discuss antenatal care with your midwife or GP.

Q **How can I arrange a home birth privately?**
A
If you wish, you can pay an independent midwife to give you total care through your pregnancy, labour and after. To find an independent midwife contact the Association of Independent Midwives (see page 193).

Being strong

You may find it difficult to arrange the birth you want. Before you start, ask yourself:

♦ Can I summon up the stamina, courage, and persistence to overcome obstacles that are likely to be put in my way?

♦ Where can I obtain the emotional support and practical help from other people that I shall need?

♦ Am I prepared to be assertive, to state what I want, avoiding both aggression and submission, and to negotiate the care that I believe is right for me and my baby?

your midwife

A midwife is quite distinct from a nurse, though midwives
have often trained as nurses before training as midwives. In
some countries, such as the Netherlands, Denmark and France,
there is "direct entry" for most midwives. They do not have
to be nurses first, but go straight into midwifery education.
In others, such as Australia, they must be nurses first. Britain
has a mix of nurse-midwives and direct entry midwives. Direct
entry ensures that a midwife's main focus is on birth as a
normal life event, rather than a disease and malfunction.

the role of midwives

There is a handful of countries with no organized midwifery system
at all: Panama, El Salvador, Venezuela, Colombia, Honduras, the
Dominican Republic, and Burundi. Alone of all Western industrialized countries, Canada has been without a legal midwifery system
of any kind until recently. But now midwifery is recognized and
professional training developed in Ontario, British Columbia,
Alberta and Manitoba.

Midwives are practitioners in their own right and are the only
people whose training is concerned solely with caring for women in
childbirth. Obstetricians are first and foremost gynaecologists, and
their status comes from this rather than from baby-catching. Any
doctor is legally allowed to deliver babies, even those with no special
training. Indeed in a modern hospital many doctors with obstetric
training have never had a chance to see a birth without intervention
of any kind, since even in straightforward labours interventions such
as artificial rupture of the membranes, withholding food and fluids
from women, and the use of intravenous drips are standard practices.
So some doctors see their involvement with childbirth as limited to
dealing with abnormalities and complications.

In some countries, such as Britain, midwives have a duty to attend a woman in childbirth when called, wherever the mother is, though they also have to obey instructions from their employers, the NHS Trust. This puts them in a difficult position. It is a woman's right to give birth where she chooses, and she does not need to book with a doctor for maternity care. Nor does she require a doctor's permission for a home birth. She, or someone else, must summon midwife help once labour is under way, or as soon as possible after the birth.

Traditional midwifery

Midwives have a long history of persecution going back to the Middle Ages, when many were burned as witches. In North America midwives who arrived in the waves of migration in the 19th century came to be dismissed as relics of an outmoded life-style and of European traditions in childbirth, on which migrants had turned their backs in favour of modern medicine. Where in the early years of the 20th century most women were cared for in their homes by midwives and family doctors, by the 1940s this had changed to hospital care by doctors, with nurses doing the minor tasks. In remote areas, where few doctors wanted to work, midwifery continued to be practised. The 1970s saw a rebirth of midwifery in North America, against strong medical opposition.

A midwife:

"The great advantage of home birth is that the labour is undisturbed. The woman does not have to be moved, and the surroundings are familiar. I don't have all the paperwork that I must do in hospital, and we are all more relaxed."

For a midwife to attend birth is in many cases against the law. It is a radical act. There is an underground midwifery, and midwives constantly risk imprisonment for practising medicine without a licence and, if a baby dies during or after birth, for manslaughter or murder. While some states now register or license midwives, in others the practice of midwifery is still a crime.

Many doctors in North America oppose midwifery because they believe it is dangerous and it threatens their profession and their incomes. They are of the opinion that midwifery offers mothers sub-standard care: "Why settle for a Ford when you can have a Cadillac?" They see themselves as the Cadillacs of birth. It is only in North America, and in hospitals elsewhere that are based on the American model, that obstetric nurses are used in place of midwives, and that the word "midwife" suggests outdated care by old grannies.

Actually, some of those granny midwives were very good. There is much we can learn from traditional midwifery in rural areas, not only in North America, but anywhere where women healers are part of a tradition of helping women through the biological transitions of their lives, and in assisting, not only at each person's coming to birth, but also giving strength and comfort at the surrendering of life.

Midwifery today

Midwives working outside hospital resort to intervention less readily than hospital midwives, because events that would be considered abnormal according to the paradigm of standard hospital labour are considered normal away from the rigid protocols of the hospital.

They are used to control people waiting in the antenatal clinic, to do menial jobs such as weighing women and putting a stick in a urine sample to note whether it changes colour, to chaperone doctors when they do a vaginal examination, to prepare equipment for the obstetrician to perform an intervention in labour and to clean up afterwards, to keep records, and in some countries where there are too many doctors – such as Italy – to be the doctor's assistant at the birth. Sweden and the Netherlands, both countries with very few baby deaths, are notable exceptions to this trend, and in each midwives have retained their professional integrity, with nearly all of the Swedish midwives working in hospitals, but most Dutch midwives doing home births.

Some midwives like being absorbed into hospital systems and do not want more responsibility. Others feel the freedom to exercise their skills has been eroded. In hospitals women are often seen by junior doctors learning about obstetrics who make decisions which might be very different from those made by an experienced midwife. She may also feel that many interventionist procedures are being carried out unnecessarily by some senior doctors and obstetricians.

A doctor:
"I have learned most about birth from midwives."

So midwives are in a difficult position. Some serve women outside hospital and attend home births and work in birth centres although, to do this, they may have to become independent, private midwives – in most countries separate from the standard health service.

In the Netherlands independent midwifery is the norm, and midwives are on a professional par with general practitioners. About 70 per cent of them work outside hospitals and 16 per cent in hospitals. (The rest are in clinics, midwifery schools, research, and so on.)

In Italy, in contrast, the vast majority work in hospitals and only a handful are independent. For most Italian women, except those in cities such as Florence, Rome, Genoa, and Turin, who are now seeking home birth in increasing numbers, it is considered a sign of poverty to go to a midwife. Find out more about independent midwives on page 193.

the midwife and home birth

For a midwife who has worked only in hospitals, it can be threatening to take on a home birth. The worst mistake is to attempt to practise exactly as she would in hospital. The midwife needs to think through how she is going to support the woman so that there is the greatest chance of labour progressing naturally at its own pace in its own way.

A midwife's responsibilities

Anxiety is contaminating. Anyone who is apprehensive around a woman in labour communicates his or her own fear, and can have a negative effect on the labour. It is the responsibility of the midwife to face up to and explore her fears in advance of attending a home birth, and to share them with colleagues who are experienced and working outside hospital, so that she does not bring infectious anxiety with her to a birth. It helps if she has already attended births outside hospital as an assistant to an experienced midwife.

When a midwife attends in quiet confidence, she is able to tolerate inaction and watch and wait on this child's coming to life, giving the mother of her own strength and inner joy.

"All midwives are based at our hospital . . . When I started labour, my husband had to go and fetch the midwives from the hospital (I suppose they were without cars). On his arrival the Night Sister greeted him with "Couldn't you persuade her to come in? It would be much safer". It was good to be at home but, if there can be such a thing, it was a hospitalized home confinement. They turned our bedroom into a hospital. Everything was timed, recorded, methodical, sterile."

Who makes a good midwife?

♦ A good midwife blends with the surroundings, merging with the pattern of that woman's life. She does not take charge or take over. She does not "manage" labour. Her task is more difficult. It demands great strength of personality. She observes minutely and with sensitive awareness everything that is occuring and is always aware of what is happening in the mind of the woman she is attending.

♦ A baby may weigh three kilos or five kilos and be of normal birth weight. In the same way a labour can be normal and yet far from average. Dilatation may be slow or rapid. The woman may have an overwhelming desire to push or almost none. Expulsion may take ten minutes or four hours. There may be lulls and rest phases. Each labour has its rhythm, its cadences, which make it different from others.

♦ A good midwife understands when she should stand back and let things unfold, and knows when to intervene. And the interventions are rare. Far more often she gives quiet, tender support to the woman, simply allowing the energy of birth to sweep through the mother's body, and helping her to find strength within herself. When you see a river in full flood, you know that you cannot fight its power. But you can use this energy so that its flow sweeps you onwards.

♦ A woman should be able to expect open and honest communication with the midwife. Instead of "reassurance" there is frank explanation, exploring of options, a genuine sharing between the two women, which goes far beyond the trite phrases that are sometimes trotted out in an attempt to keep a patient docile and placid.

When a woman and her midwife relate to each other with mutual respect, warmth, and openness, it is as if they are on a journey in which exciting discoveries are made, their understanding deepens, and they are both enriched by the birth experience.

♦ A good midwife loves women. She does not dominate, direct, or even instruct. The word "midwife" is Anglo-Saxon for "with woman". The midwife is side by side and with the woman. Except on the rare occasions when she needs to take decisive action to avert danger, she follows rather than leads. Ina May Gaskin, spiritual midwife at The Farm, the alternative-style community in Tennessee, says, "Pregnant and birthing mothers are elemental forces, in the same way that gravity, thunderstorms, earthquakes and hurricanes are elemental forces. In order to understand the laws of their energy flow, you have to love and respect them for their magnificence, at the same time that you study them with the accuracy of a true scientist."*

♦ A good midwife does not criticize or judge the woman, and even though a woman may be submissive and seek approval, she helps her to stand on her own feet and find the locus of control inside herself.

When women give birth in hospital, they often apologize to their midwives. Professor Mavis Kirkham wrote of a hospital research project, "Most of the women I observed in labour apologized. Many

apologized frequently if they felt they were not behaving well or were "being a nuisance", or "causing trouble" by making requests or simply receiving routine care from busy staff. The commonest words I heard women say immediately after delivery were "I'm sorry . . ."*
When women placate authority, their deference is implicit acknowledgement of an institutional power structure in which they are the lowest level. They are intruders on the professional territory of the hospital. If midwives accept these apologies, they too acknowledge and submit to this power structure.

♦ A good midwife is not only someone who delivers a baby. She is midwife to a woman's transformation to motherhood and a man's transformation to fatherhood. She is midwife to all the dreams and hopes surrounding the coming to being of that child, and to the process of maturing and growth that is involved for both parents.

Meeting your midwife

Even though midwifery is the foundation of care in childbirth throughout Europe, and the system would collapse if midwives walked out, most countries no longer provide continuity in care. Different groups of midwives work in the antenatal clinic, the labour and delivery rooms, and on the postpartum ward. At a time in their lives when women are most vulnerable, they meet strangers. In Britain attempts are being made – through the creation of midwife teams who get to know the mothers during pregnancy – to deal with this problem, which is frustrating and often confusing for midwives as well as mothers. But only in Denmark and the Netherlands is it the norm to have continuity of care from your own midwife. In southern Europe doctors have totally taken over antenatal care, and even in countries where midwife care at birth is the normal system, a woman having her baby in hospital may never meet the midwives assigned to her until she is admitted in labour. Having your baby outside hospital may be your only opportunity to get to know your midwife.

"As a midwife I would never persuade a woman to have a home birth. She's got to be very sure that it's what she wants. But I am certain that the majority of complications arise purely because women are in hospital."

Questions to ask

At your first meetings with the midwife, or with the small group of midwives who are attending you, there will be many questions to ask. If you are choosing an independent midwife, you will need to put these questions before you can come to a firm arrangement with

The role of the midwife

One of the most important questions of all for you to answer is whether you like her as a person and feel relaxed and confident with her. Can you be completely open about how you feel and what you want? Talk with other women for whom she has cared to find out about their experience with her. You can learn a great deal from them.

Points to consider

You may want to discuss these issues with your midwife:

♦ Nutrition in pregnancy

♦ Who you would like with you at the birth

♦ Fetal monitoring

♦ Moving around during labour

♦ Positions for birth

♦ Using a birth pool

♦ Exactly what help she gives a mother to avoid the need for episiotomy

♦ Her basic beliefs about birth and breastfeeding

♦ What exactly you are hoping for with this birth

Q A How are midwives different from obstetricians?

Unlike obstetricians, the main focus of the care they offer is the normal, not the pathological, and the whole woman rather than one organ, the uterus. A good midwife knows how to keep birth normal.

Q A What does a midwife do?

The midwife is a specialist in childbearing, qualified to take responsibility for women antenatally, through the birth itself, and for four weeks afterwards. She has specific skills to support the physiological process, understands deviations from the normal, and knows when obstetric advice or assistance is required.

Q A How is this different in a hospital?

Hospital midwives often become subordinate members of teams headed by obstetricians, and have been powerless to prevent this. Some opt for the security in a hospital system and do not step out of line. Others fight that system from the inside.

each other. Either way, you won't want to fire questions at her, but can incorporate many of these into your discussion with her:

♦ How long have you been a midwife?

♦ Why did you become a midwife?

♦ What was your training?

♦ How many mothers have you attended, and of these how many were home births or not in a large hospital?

♦ Do you work with other midwives?

♦ What happens if two women are in labour at the same time?

♦ Will I be able to meet your colleagues?

♦ What is your back-up system? Do you work with any doctors?

♦ What equipment do you carry with you? Do you carry any drugs for pain relief and to stimulate the uterus?

♦ What resuscitation equipment for the baby do you carry?

♦ What antenatal care do you provide? Are there any home visits?

♦ Do you offer childbirth classes or pregnancy discussion groups? If not, what classes do you recommend?

♦ What postnatal care do you provide?

♦ What do you do if a woman has a very long labour?

♦ What will happen if transfer to hospital should be necessary?

♦ Why would you transfer; what are your transfer rates?

♦ If she works in a birth centre or GP unit: Are there any standard procedures, such as compulsory fetal monitoring, birth positions, and so on?

♦ What are your views on routine episiotomy? What is your episiotomy rate?

♦ What is your rate for an intact perineum?

♦ What happens if my perineum needs suturing? Will you do this or call a doctor?

♦ When are your holidays? If you are away and I go into labour, whom should I call?

♦ For an independent midwife, ask her fee, when it should be paid, and what is included.

"She was wonderful . . . She visited me at home in the early stages of my pregnancy, and chatted as a friend would over a cup of coffee . . . As my pregnancy progressed, she called at the house once a week for her own personal check-up. She made friends with my three-year-old, letting her feel my tummy and listen to the baby's heartbeat."

A woman who becomes a midwife cares deeply for women and loves babies. Yet hospital midwives often learn to guard their feelings and have been forced to hold back from giving themselves completely. They have been warned not to "become emotionally involved". When a midwife works in an environment outside the hospital system, she is free to be herself and to have a close, caring relationship with a woman whom she comes to know, not as a patient, but as a sister.

A midwife's visit

For any woman who only meets her midwife when she is
admitted to hospital in labour, and who then may find that this
person disappears with the next shift change, the experience of
bearing a child is bound to be fragmented and depersonalized.
When a woman gets to know her midwife during pregnancy
and the two become friends, a bond of understanding develops,
and the emotional support the midwife gives can help the
mother feel confident and strong.

It is fun for the
older child too. He
learns about how
babies are born in
the most natural
way possible, is
shown how to feel
the firm curve of
the baby's bottom,
and is delighted
when a little foot
kicks against his
hand. The new
baby will not come
as a surprise or as
an alien invader, but
is someone whom
he has already
learned about and
even touched.

The midwife fixes the blood
pressure cuff and starts to blow
it up. The child is intrigued as
she explains it, and then enjoys
having a go himself. This kind
of relationship with a child is
much easier when antenatal
care takes place at home, so that
the older child is in a familiar
environment and on his own
ground, and the midwife comes
as a friend of the family.

getting ready

Now that you have made the decision to give birth out of hospital, you can prepare to make it the best experience possible. The chances of a safe, happy birth are enormously increased if you approach labour healthy, energetic, well-nourished, and self-confident, and if you learn movements that allow your body to open up, and know how to relax and breathe rhythmically.

your antenatal care

The fragmentation of care that often occurs in hospital clinics results from different staff members performing different tests as women are shuffled from one line of chairs to another, from room to room, and cubicle to cubicle. Yet, if you escape being screened by a variety of anonymous doctors, nurses, midwives and radiographers, you are still not receiving good care if you have tests that detract from, or take the place of, your caregivers' relationship with you as a unique human being. Antenatal care should be far more than screening for abnormalities. You need holistic care, to be cared for as a whole person, rather than merely tested for potential problems.

"I have to go on the bus to get to the clinic, as I haven't a car. The journey takes 45 minutes each way, and I usually have to wait at least half an hour. I have two – perhaps three – minutes with the doctor. The only reason I go is because I'd worry that something was going wrong if I didn't."

Even if a woman has only one caregiver, or a small group of caregivers, the medical model is often adopted. It entails turning her into a patient and dividing up information about her body so that it can be laid out on a record card: blood pressure, weight, urine, haemoglobin, and height of fundus. Her hopes and fears, the stresses of her daily life, financial worries, family conflicts, work problems, are seen as irrelevant compared with physical symptoms that can be checked, enumerated, and recorded.

Many unnecessary investigations take place in antenatal clinics today. Some are potentially harmful. Since the early years of the last century, when obstetric-style antenatal care was first introduced, tests have proliferated. Doctors seem to be under the impression that any item of information might come in useful sometime. But information is useless unless it affects the kind of care that is provided.

Midwives in traditional cultures were giving antenatal care long before the 20th century, visiting the pregnant woman's home to teach her about pregnancy, to discuss diet, work, and exercise, to massage her with oil and palpate her uterus, to talk with her about her husband and family, to ward off danger with shared religious rites and prayers, and to make plans for the birth. Traditional midwives have usually been far more involved with birth than simply acting as birth attendants.

Today obstetricians construct the agenda for antenatal care. As we have seen already, there is strong evidence that other influences on pregnant women – socio-economic conditions that result in inequalities in health – usually have more effect on the outcome of pregnancy than anything that the most dedicated of obstetricians can do in an antenatal clinic. Socially deprived women, who are most in need of care, are most likely to delay seeking it. A woman with a ten-month-old baby and a two-and-a-half-year-old child, no help at home, nobody else to care for the children, and no private transport, may find it difficult to attend an antenatal clinic even though it is only two or three miles away. A teenager who is hoping against hope that she is not pregnant, trying to hide it from her family, and with no idea of how to get help, is unlikely to find her way to the antenatal clinic until pregnancy is well-advanced.

It is much safer to have a baby if you are educated and well-off than if you are uneducated and poor. In England and

"He said, "The baby's very small, you know. Try and eat more." Next time I saw another doctor, who told me, "You've got a good-sized baby there. It's going to be a whopper!" I don't know what to believe. Should I be stuffing myself to try and make the baby bigger or will it be so huge that it can't get out?"

"It was a shambles really. The doctor gave me the wrong card. It was a different blood group, and it said "Rhesus negative" but I am Rhesus positive. I didn't realize till much later, but I could have had a whole lot of treatment I didn't need, and the other woman, who had my card, wouldn't have had treatment that she needed. At least they let us keep our own records. If the clinic had kept them, it might never have been found out."

"The midwife came to see me at home and spent a lot of time talking about what I wanted. She became a friend and we all look forward to her visits."

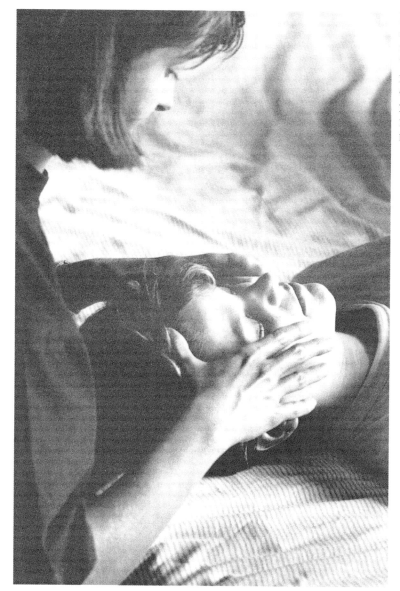

Learning the art of massage – touch that helps you "centre down" in your body, is one of the skills that you and your partner can practise together.

Wales, perinatal mortality rates are worked out on the basis of the husband's occupation. Twice as many babies die in social class 5, at the bottom of the scale, as in social class 1, at the top .*

Standard antenatal care entails up to 15 visits to a clinic or hospital, or a mixture of both, and a woman may encounter 50 or more different professionals, many of whom make conflicting comments and give contradictory advice. Far from providing reassurance, these encounters increase anxiety.

Routine antenatal tests

There is no point in having tests unless their results are going to affect care. Useless information provided by routine tests is often employed as a charm against a perilous passage, in the same way that talismans have been used traditionally by pregnant women to guard against evil. With modern antenatal care this information is often not even conveyed to the mother, but is retained by the doctor and recorded, as part of a series of illegible hieroglyphs resembling mystic runes, in case-notes that are sometimes not even passed on to other caregivers.

The results of most tests have a margin of error that is often wide and can lead to false negative and false positive diagnoses. False negative diagnosis suggests that there is no problem when in fact there is one. False positive diagnosis appears to reveal a problem when there is none. Both are dangerous. The first gives rise to complacency in the face of special risk. The second causes needless anxiety, and may lead to unnecessary interventions, such as induction of labour or Caesarean section.

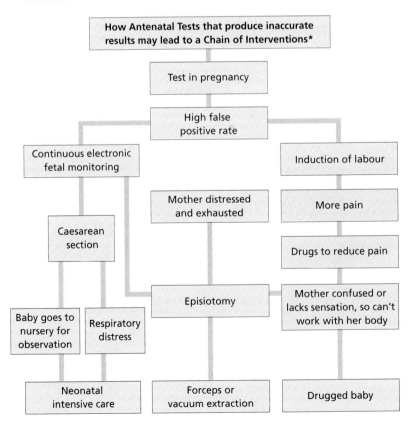

♦ There is nothing gained from regularly testing urine for sugar in pregnancy unless you are diabetic. A trace of sugar in urine is very common. It may simply mean that you have recently eaten something especially sweet. Bananas sometimes have this effect.

♦ Routine weighing is a waste of time too. Weight checks give useful information only if you started pregnancy very underweight or very overweight. The baby's growth is better assessed by having one or two caregivers regularly palpate your uterus so that they are in touch, literally, with the baby's development.

♦ Vaginal examinations in pregnancy are usually unnecessary. In some countries, including the USA, they are performed weekly starting at 37 weeks. In Britain one vaginal examination is often done routinely some time between 33 and 37 weeks. However, vaginal examinations increase the risk of infection and premature rupture of the membranes and, because of this, Caesarean section.*

♦ Ultrasound enables obstetricians to visualize the baby in the uterus and learn much more about fetal development, and it reveals certain abnormalities. If you have a scan at around 16 weeks, the date of conception, and hence the expected date of delivery, can be estimated fairly accurately, but only within two weeks. If you are unsure about the date you conceived, you might decide that this is a good reason for choosing to have a scan. If you have already had a low-birth-weight baby, you may also want to monitor fetal growth with several ultrasound scans. Diagnosis of the baby's weight based on fundal height is almost as accurate as that from ultrasound, so whether or not you have a series of scans is up to you.*

♦ Biochemical tests of fetal wellbeing proliferated in the 70s and 80s. They included alpha-feta-protein testing, measurement of HCG (human chorionic gonadotrophin), placental proteins, HPL (human placental lactogen) and oestrogen levels with 24-hour urine specimens, blood tests, or, occasionally, measurement of levels in the saliva. A small proportion of the biochemical tests available can be useful in early pregnancy to screen for abnormalities. But tests later in pregnancy to try to predict low birth weight, premature birth, or stillbirth are a waste of time.*

♦ Cardiotocography – fetal heart-rate monitoring in pregnancy – has added to obstetricians' knowledge about life inside the uterus, but four randomized controlled trials have not demonstrated any direct benefit for mothers and babies. So you may decide that it is not worth having this.*

Holistic antenatal care

If you are having holistic antenatal care, you will be offered only those screening procedures that are likely to give useful information and make a difference in the care that is given during pregnancy or at the birth. While being alert to the possibility of pathology, its main focus is woman-centred.

A holistic approach enables you to care for yourself, instead of just being at the receiving end of care. It is concerned with feelings and relationships that are important to you rather than merely with physiology. And it helps you to grow in self-awareness, self-confidence, and strength. Holistic antenatal care is empowering.

For care to be holistic, it is essential to have a continuing relationship with a few caregivers only, who get to know you well and who make time at each visit to obtain full and accurate information, and to talk freely, in a totally accepting atmosphere. There is genuine sharing.

what is the best kind of diet in pregnancy?

When you conceive, and in the first 8 weeks of pregnancy, it is important to have a diet rich in folic acid. This is present in dark green leafy vegetables, whole grains, yeast and nuts. It is in liver, too, but it is easy to get too much Vitamin A from liver and that is toxic. It is a good idea to take supplementary folic acid if you are likely to get pregnant and in early pregnancy when rapid cell division is taking place and the baby's spinal cord and brain is forming.

Everything you eat during pregnancy should enhance your feeling of wellbeing and be good for you and the baby. Choose wholegrain bread and cereals, fruit and vegetables – freshly picked whenever you can get them – and to ensure a good supply of vitamin C have one raw fruit or vegetable meal every day. Eat some protein at each meal, either in the form of meat, fish, dairy products (such as cheese, milk, eggs – thoroughly cooked – and yogurt), a soya bean product such as tofu, or a mix of pulses (peas, beans or lentils) and grains (bread, rice or pasta). Eat iron-rich foods: leafy green vegetables and egg yolks are good sources. Use olive oil, sunflower oil and other polyunsaturated oils as a large proportion of your fat intake, and enjoy the sugar found naturally in fresh and dried fruit, rather than adding sugar to desserts.

An excess of any one food type is bad. It is possible to have carrot poisoning, and to die of it. People have had coronaries associated with eating, among other things, excessive meat and dairy foods.

When considering your diet in pregnancy, think about the foods you enjoy most. It may be a good idea to write them down. Then look at what you have written to see if any of them do not measure up to your standards of nutrition. Are there any junk foods? Do they contain artificial colourings or are they full of preservatives? Do any provide empty calories? Are there too many fatty foods? If you are particularly fond of food which you know is not good for you, you might then list what you especially like about it: salty, crunchy, crisp, sweet, smooth, filling, quick to make, cheap, reminds me of home (or Rome, or Vienna, or somewhere else). Invariably, there are alternatives that bring a similar sense of wellbeing.

When you look at what you enjoy about the foods that are not so good for you, think how you can find the same qualities in more nutritious foods. If you want an instant food, choose nuts and raisins, bite into a banana or apple, or bake a potato in the microwave. If you long for something hot and satisfying, home-made soup is more nutritious, and probably tastier and more satisfying than a mug of hot chocolate (though you need not rule out the hot chocolate entirely).

At the end of pregnancy many women become constipated, and this can be treated by eating more wholegrain bread and muesli. But this is effective only if you also cut your fat intake to the minimum.

Salt in pregnancy

Despite the advice often given to omit salt in order to prevent pre-eclampsia, there is no convincing evidence that salt restriction is effective in achieving this. A study of 2,000 pregnant women, half of whom were recommended to increase salt, and the other half to avoid it, revealed that there were significantly fewer women with pre-eclampsia in the high-salt group.* Nor do you need to force yourself to eat large quantities of high-protein foods, since an excessive amount of protein can reduce a baby's birth weight.*

In an overview of all the studies of nutrition in pregnancy, the head of the epidemiology programme at the Human Nutrition Research Center on Ageing at Tuft's University in Massachusetts concludes: "There can be no rational justification for either allowing pregnant women to go hungry or for imposing either dietary restrictions or marked manipulation of the dietary constituents upon them."* So relax and enjoy your food!

medication

You will know already that it is wise to avoid drugs in pregnancy unless you really need them. But there can be few hard and fast rules, and it is usually a question of weighing up the risks and benefits of the drug against the risks and benefits of not treating a disease. Sometimes a pregnant woman has an illness that holds possible dangers for the baby. Then treating the illness is a sensible choice, even though it entails taking a drug. A high fever, for example, can cause miscarriage and, if the fever can't be brought down in any other way, it is probably better to take some paracetamol.

All dietary supplements, including vitamins and minerals, are drugs and may overload the system with one mineral or vitamin and result in nutritional deficiency. Some supplements – such as vitamins A and D – are toxic in high doses. So avoid mega-vitamins and, unless you know that you suffer from nutritional deficiencies that cannot be rectified by a change of diet, do not take supplementary vitamins and minerals, other than folic acid and other B vitamins.

Herbs

A drug is not necessarily safe for pregnancy because it occurs naturally in the wild. Herbs can be powerful, and they, too, may be poisonous. Most herbs prescribed by reputable herbalists – select one who is a member of an association of registered practitioners of alternative or complementary medicine – are safe. But others that may be teratogenic (causing congenital malformation) or lead to miscarriage. The following herbs are potentially dangerous for anyone, whether pregnant or not: comfrey, berberis, ragwort, prickly ash, excessive intake of ginseng, feverfew, and the kernels of apricots, plums, and peaches.

Some herbs increase uterine muscle tone, so can be helpful in producing effective contractions in labour. But the same herbs used in pregnancy, in high doses and by women who are particularly vulnerable, may be associated with miscarriage. So it is wise to avoid herbs such as feverfew and pennyroyal.*

Supplements

If you are healthy, you are unlikely to need iron supplements. An increased blood supply in pregnancy results in dilution of haemoglobin, and this often causes a normal drop in haemoglobin. This is a natural process that helps the flow of blood across the placenta, in fact it is a sign of fetal well being. If your haemoglobin level does not fall beneath 11 grams per decilitre, there is no need for iron supplements.* Unnecessary iron supplementation can cause constipation that results in piles, and may result in macrocytosis, where red blood cells enlarge and become sticky so that they cannot flow through fine capillaries, impairing circulation.

Very high haemoglobin levels in pregnancy are associated with low birth weight. So there is a disadvantage in artificially boosting your haemoglobin level unless you are anaemic.*

It is in the interest of pharmaceutical companies who manufacture vitamin and mineral supplements to sell them as widely as possible and to persuade doctors that their patients need them. There is no reason why any pregnant woman should be dosed with these as a matter of routine, and vitamins and minerals are best obtained from a well-balanced diet with plenty of fresh fruit and vegetables, wholegrain cereals, and protein in the form of milk and milk products, pulses, and – for non-vegetarians – meat and fish.

When a woman's haemoglobin is low, caregivers are concerned that if she loses much blood in childbirth she will be very weak and ill, and need a blood transfusion. This is one reason why, when haemoglobin levels are low at the end of pregnancy, they may be reluctant to support her wish to have a home birth. It seems sensible to have a blood test, at, say, 36 weeks to check the haemoglobin level, so that there is time for any supplementation to take effect, if it is needed. If a woman is still anaemic when labour starts, the third stage can be actively managed with an injection of Syntometrine. This reduces blood loss and makes haemhorrage

You can devise your own exercise and relaxation routines. Many public pools offer women-only sessions.

Yoga

support you in different positions during labour.

Q **Does it have any other effects?**

A

Yoga and active birth classes also lead to improved physical co-ordination, increased self-confidence, and a sense of inner balance.

Q **Is yoga safe for pregnant women?**

A

Special yoga classes for pregnancy should be safe, but if any movement proves a strain or causes pain, drop it from the routine, and concentrated on easy, flowing, rhythmic movements instead.

Q **Must I have done yoga before?**

A

Many classes designed for pregnant women are suitable for complete beginners. Always check this when you book the class.

Q **How can yoga help in pregnancy?**

A

Special yoga classes for pregnancy are useful, since they include opening movements for the pelvis and, at the same time, help you to find a focus of concentration inside yourself in a very satisfying way. Yoga also teaches you to breathe rhythmically and fully.

Q **Can yoga actually help me in labour?**

A

Yes. Many active birth classes are based on yoga. In these you learn movements to enable muscles to "give" and help your pelvis widen to let the baby through, practise a range of upright positions and movements and discover how your partner can

Q **When can I start yoga classes?**

A

You can attend classes from when you are three months pregnant, but again, check this with your yoga teacher.

less likely. A midwife at a home birth will feel far more confident if she knows that you are willing to accept this option if she considers it necessary.

exercise

Taking a form of regular exercise that you really enjoy helps you to feel positive about your pregnant body, tones your muscles, and whips up your circulation.

♦ Swimming is an excellent form of exercise to take in pregnancy, because it is so easy to move when floating in water that takes your weight.

♦ Brisk walking in the countryside or a park is good too.

♦ Many women go to aerobic classes which are specially adapted to pregnancy.

♦ One form of dancing is especially suitable: belly dancing – the slow, sinuous kind, rather than rapid gyrations with a diamond in your navel! Belly dancing was taught traditionally in North Africa as part of fertility rituals to mark a girl's passage to womanhood, and women attending a birth danced while the mother rolled her pelvis in a similar way during contractions. Any movement like this that frees the pelvis can help the baby's head to rotate and descend deep into the pelvis.

♦ Yoga classes can be helpful, both as a form of exercise and to help you relax.

One of the best things about exercise is the healthy glow and sense of luxurious relaxation that comes afterwards. Give yourself time to enjoy that.

Exercise to avoid

♦ Competitive games, in which you are inclined to ignore the messages of tiredness and pain coming from your body because you are out to beat the other person, are not a good idea in pregnancy so should be avoided.

♦ If your pelvic ligaments stretch too much in late pregnancy, so that you feel like a disjointed doll, have backache, and stumble often, pronounced movements of the pelvis that entail hollowing the lower part of your back may make the situation worse. You should select only those movements that involve tightening your buttocks and abdominal muscles, gently releasing, and then tightening them again.

♦ Remember that if any movement in an exercise class proves a strain or causes you pain, you should drop it from your routine immediately, and concentrate on making easy, flowing, rhythmic movements instead.

rest and relaxation

You will get the most out of your pregnancy if you can take time to rest and nurture yourself. That means making a space in your life to do anything you like – to listen to music, to read, to dream or to do nothing at all – a space free from the stress of striving to reach a goal, to live up to a standard, or to please someone else.

It is very difficult to do this when you have other children and little or no help with them, difficult to do if your partner dismisses domestic work as trivial and something he was never much good at anyway, and difficult if your job is the kind which consumes all your energy. Your own feelings of responsibility, and the guilt you feel when you are not meeting other people's expectations of you, may hold you back from creating this small, private citadel of time and space that is yours alone. But if you can do it, you will feel more "centred" and better able to relax and enjoy being pregnant.

I remember reading a short story in which the heroine was in labour: ""I must. I MUST relax!" she muttered fiercely." The feeling that relaxation is compulsory, that if you don't manage to relax, something awful will happen, and that you have to fight to achieve it makes you more tense. Relaxation is a luxury.

If you are having your baby at home or in another out-of-hospital setting, relaxation is the basis of your preparation for birth. It is also a major protection against stress in pregnancy, and is invaluable after the baby comes, when you need to relax in order to breastfeed, as well as to make all the adjustments – the amazing leap across the great divide – entailed in becoming a parent.

Creating a relaxing environment

It helps to have a quiet, peaceful place where you are least likely to be interrupted, and where, like an animal in her lair, you can go to ground. It might be your bed, the bath, a garden, a couch in front of an open fire, at the seashore or in a meadow. Any comfortable space where, if only for ten minutes, you will not be disturbed by the phone ringing or people demanding your attention, will do well.

First make a nest for yourself with cushions, perhaps a duvet, a beanbag, or some rolled-up towels or rugs. When you are in the bath, slip a small rolled towel behind your neck or use a Chinese neck cushion for support. If you are in a chair, on the ground, or in bed, either recline, well-supported with cushions, or lie down on your side.

In late pregnancy avoid lying flat on your back. Your heavy uterus tends to press on the vena cava, the large vein in the lower part of your body, when you are lying in this position. This slows down the blood flow back to your heart and may make you feel sick and giddy, as well as restricting blood flow to the placenta, and oxygen to the baby. So, either sitting well-propped-up or lying on your side, support your head and neck with cushions and get comfortable. If you are on your side, a cushion under your upper knee often helps. If sitting up, you will need one in the small of your back. The first few times you do this, it is useful to have someone read the following passage for you, slowly, in a low-pitched voice.

Bend your arms and knees and let your body spread, taking as much space as possible. Release tension on a long breath out. Then let the breath flow in when you are ready for it. Don't suck air in. Just allow your lungs to fill. There is a slight pause, as when the crest of a wave is reached, after which you give another breath out, relaxing all down your back and right down to your toes as you do so.

As you listen to the sound of your breathing, be aware of your whole body: your skin where it touches the air and the fabric of your clothing, the strong muscles underneath, your swelling uterus with the baby moving inside it, and the blood pulsing through your body.

Are there any parts of your body that are holding on to tension? You may want to find a more comfortable position. Roll your head slightly forwards and round your shoulders. If you are not completely comfortable, have a stretch and re-settle. Or roll into a ball like a hedgehog, and then slowly uncurl until you feel at ease.

As you continue, listen to your slow breathing and relax a little more with each breath out. Enjoy your breathing as if you were listening to waves on the seashore. Focus on the breath out, and you will find that the breath in looks after itself.

To derive the most advantage from relaxation, you should practise it daily, setting aside a regular time for this self-nurturing. If you have the opportunity, take a rest after lunch, or perhaps at some point in the evening. But, even if you can do it only when you wake in the morning or go to bed at night, or if you wake to empty your bladder and find it difficult to get back to sleep, ten minutes' relaxation will help you.

should I do breathing exercises?

You will know how to breathe when you are in labour, just as you know how to breathe now.

Breathing responds instantly to emotions. When we are feeling apprehensive, we breathe jerkily. We hold our breath if we are very afraid, and pain can make us gasp. Under stress some people breathe heavily and quickly, and hyperventilate. The sensations of hyperventilation are pins and needles in the fingers, numbness around the mouth, and a feeling of dizziness and sickness. Giving birth, even the most beautiful and satisfying birth, is a highly stressful activity, so it is understandable that many women over-breathe and hyperventilate when the contractions are coming thick and fast.

Getting prepared

During your pregnancy get to know your breathing habits, noticing how your breathing changes with your emotions. If this is difficult to observe, ask your partner to help. Are there times when you breathe arrhythmically, hold your breath, or over breathe?

Tension in breathing usually stems from the shoulders. Drop your shoulders and you will find that you are able to breathe more easily. Whenever you are aware of being under stress, breathe out, drop your shoulders, and relax. Your breathing will respond immediately and become rhythmic and even. Breathing should not be hard work!

When you take the time to relax, notice how you are breathing. Breathe smoothly and slowly so that it feels as if you are breathing down into your pelvis and touching your baby with each breath you take. When your breathing is relaxed, your baby often becomes quite active.

Breathing in labour

During labour, long slow breaths will help at the onset and the end of every contraction. You may be able to breathe like this right through a contraction too. But many women feel the need to breathe more quickly as contractions become more powerful and are closer together. If this is how it is for you, let your breathing speed up and at the same time make it lighter. Rapid deep breathing will result in hyperventilation. Rapid light breathing at the height of contractions can help you scale the peaks.

When contractions are at their strongest, it is impossible to move the abdominal wall or to feel anything in your pelvis other than their power. The tightening of longitudinal muscle fibres results in a lifting of the abdominal wall, because the contraction causes the top of the uterus, the fundus, to tilt forwards, so there is a great swelling that also presses against the diaphragm. From your diaphragm down, you feel as if you are all one huge contraction. Let your breathing "dance" above this and breathe through parted lips with the tip of your tongue resting against your lower teeth. Have sips of water or ice to suck in the spaces between contractions, so that your mouth does not get dry. Avoid huffing and puffing. The breath should be as light as a whisper. Then, as the contraction reaches its climax and starts to fade, you can form slow, full breaths again. It is important not to forget to do this. You and your baby will welcome the extra oxygen as each contraction finishes. And the slow breathing will help you relax completely in the trough between the great waves of contractions, so that you are refreshed and strong for the next one.

Taught breathing

Breathing is often taught in antenatal classes as a set of exercises, and sometimes these are very rigid and mechanical. It may be that when a woman is giving birth on alien territory, in a hospital where she is not sure what will happen, or what she will be allowed to do, such precise techniques are helpful as a distraction from pain and from an environment she sees as threatening. The exercises keep her concentrated on something she can do to help herself. I have seen women with their eyes fixed on a crack in the ceiling breathing desperately, as if clinging to a safety rope above a precipice, mentally cut off from their surroundings, unable to hear what anyone is saying, out of touch with help that is being offered. When breathing is used like this, it becomes a barrier against the environment.

You will not need to use breathing exercises if you are having your baby at home, or in an out-of-hospital setting where your attendants are friends, and where there is no need to fear intrusion.

Breathing your baby out

When your cervix is wide open and your body ready for the baby to be pushed down, your breathing changes, often dramatically. There is an involuntarily held breath that starts as a catch in the throat. This is a sign that the baby is well on its journey to birth and that you can help it out. While you can continue to breathe, you should do so. Do not attempt to hold your breath deliberately, as this forces the pace of the baby's progress and causes unnecessary stress on your pelvic floor muscles and perineum.

Then, when you get an irresistible desire to push, drop your jaw, and let yourself open up, and then begin to breathe again as soon as the urge passes.

The baby's head will press deeper and deeper until you feel it bulging against your perineum like a grapefruit. You can put your hand down and touch it. From this point on, it is important to breathe your baby out, so that you push only when you cannot resist it. Your uterus will do the work for you. Breathing through your open, relaxed mouth, in long sighs, will help your perineum relax and unfold as the baby's head oozes through.

The head is born and rotates. You look down and have the first glimpse of your baby's profile. Then the shoulders slide through and, often in one quick movement, like a fish leaping, the whole body emerges, to reveal your slippery, warm, wriggling, wonderful baby.

tuning in to your baby

When a woman does not wish professional caregivers to take over in childbirth, to manage her labour actively and make decisions without consulting her, it is important that she is in touch with her own feelings, with her body and the drama that is unfolding in it, and also with her baby. This little person is carried on the same waves of energy that sweep through her to the shores of life, sharing the experience with her.

The relationship with your baby starts long before your child is born, long before the very first contractions that herald labour. It has its tentative beginnings as soon as you are aware that you may have conceived, and ripens as you "listen" to your child's movements and conduct a two-way conversation with the world outside and the one within you. When you are in touch with your baby in the uterus, birth is only one stage in the development of a relationship that is already a reality.

A baby does not suddenly spring into action at birth. For some time before the event your baby has been a complex, coordinated human being who is already learning and communicating.

The power of touch

Babies react to touch very early, though at first this is merely a reflex response. By the time you are 12 weeks pregnant the baby is already kicking, but you do not feel it at this stage, because he or she is still too small. You usually feel movements for the first time between 17 and 20 weeks. They are like bubbles popping or minnows darting about. But even before that the baby can make complicated foot movements, twisting the foot round, curling and uncurling the toes, and "treading water".

"This child seems to understand laughter or, if we are all shouting and laughing, it starts kicking rhythmically. It touches with its feet anything placed over my abdomen. It feels like delicate exploring. There is an interval during which the baby must be locating the sensation, then a light kick in exactly the right spot."

At 16 weeks the baby reaches out with tiny hands, feeling the surrounding water, and exploring the space around and the springy walls of the uterus.

Ultrasound scanning reveals that babies often suck their thumbs, so pleasure from non-nutritive sucking is already well-established while the baby is in the uterus. It assists the coordination of sucking and swallowing necessary for feeding. All the movements that the baby makes have the effect of toning its muscles, in the same way that regular exercise undertaken by adults results in muscular development and strengthening.

what position is my baby in?

In the last few weeks of pregnancy you will probably be able to tell the position your baby is in by tracking the legs and trunk with your fingers. When your midwife or doctor palpates your uterus, he or she feels for the baby's head first, but for you it is easier to start by feeling for the feet, which may be so clearly defined that you feel you could almost measure the baby for shoes. Starting from where you can find a vigorous little foot, pass your fingers along the legs to the baby's pointed bottom, and then finally feel down the long curve of the back.

If you are giving birth out of hospital, it will help to know if your baby is head down, if the head is engaged in your pelvis, and whether the baby's back is towards your front with the head tucked forwards on the chest. When this is the case, you can be increasingly confident that the birth will be straightforward.

When the baby is head down (in the vertex or cephalic position), you feel the kicking in the upper part of the uterus. When the baby's head is up, you feel the hard ball of the head under your ribs, although you may be deceived by a big baby who is lying head-down with its bottom positioned high under your ribs.

Once the head is engaged, your diaphragm can swing down more easily than before as you take a deep breath. When your bladder is full, the head may cause pressure against it so that you want to empty your bladder often, as in the first weeks of pregnancy. This is one sign that the head is deep in the pelvis. Another is an occasional tingling in your vagina. The baby may be using your pelvic floor muscles as a trampoline, giving you short, sharp buzzing sensations like tiny electric shocks. These are a sign that the baby is in a very good position.

When the baby is curled into a ball with the back facing towards your front (in the anterior position), your navel protrudes and you can trace a firm, melon-shaped arc at the front. This is the baby's back. You will also be able to feel kicking at one side or the other under your ribs. Kicking occurs at the side opposite the baby's back.

If the baby is not yet anterior, you feel kicking all over your front, and there is a saucer-shaped dip around your navel. This suggests that the baby is posterior, with its back towards your spine. Strong contractions will be needed to turn the baby round into the ideal position for birth. Welcome them when they come, and prepare for a long first stage whilst your uterus does this work. You may have a backache labour, because the hard back of the baby's head is pressed into the small of your back. Discuss with your caregivers and birth partner how you are going to handle that.

Breech baby

If your baby is still not head down in the last weeks, you can try a pelvic tilt to shift the baby's bottom up out of your pelvis and enable him or her to somersault and turn head down. You will need to get your head lower than your pelvis, either by lying with your pelvis propped up over a couple of firm floor cushions or a beanbag with your head on the floor, or by supporting your pelvis on a low divan bed and leaning over the side of it. Lie turned towards your front rather than your back, as the baby will probably find it easier to move against your abdominal wall than against your spine. Make as much space as possible for your baby to move by ensuring that your knees are well apart and are not pressing against your abdomen. Now try moving your pelvis to encourage the baby to shift. Rolling and rocking movements are good. This is more likely to be effective at a time when you know the baby is awake and on the move. Although this may not be a posture you would choose for relaxation, once you are reasonably comfortable, relax and give long, slow, full breaths into your pelvis and release your abdominal muscles with each breath out.

Some babies somersault, but then turn back soon afterwards. Others refuse to budge at all. But, if your baby is still breech at the end of pregnancy, it is a manoeuvre worth trying for about 15 minutes, two or three times a day.

how do I make a birth plan?

Discussing your ideas about birth with whoever will attend you in labour helps you to focus your mind on what is most important to you, and enables your midwife or doctor to understand your needs.

In hospital, birth plans are often presented by anxious women, who are afraid that they will not be consulted about what is done to them during childbirth, to professionals who often feel threatened by them. I have actually heard a birth plan described by an obstetrician as "a weapon used to manipulate the professionals" and by a psychotherapist as "a transitional object", like a security blanket.

"'Birth plan?' said the doctor. "What do you want?" I began to explain. "What kind of things do you want to avoid, lovey?" she asked. I said I was not too keen on an episiotomy. She was absorbed in her own calculations. Suddenly she informed me that I was to be admitted straight away, as the baby had not grown in a fortnight. Labour might be induced that very afternoon. So much for my birth plan."

One woman's birth plan

I should like to:

♦ Walk around for as long as I like.
♦ Stand or squat during contractions.
♦ Find out for myself the easiest and most comfortable position when pushing.

♦ Have the comforting presence of a close friend, who has two children herself.
♦ Have the same midwife present throughout, one who has given me antenatal care, whom I trust, and with whom I have a personal relationship.
♦ Have no drugs.

When you are having your baby out of hospital, a birth plan is a valuable element in the communication between you and your caregivers, part of the developing relationship with them. It ought to be like this in hospital too, but often isn't. Another problem with hospital birth plans is that, although you may be encouraged to make a plan, the person with whom you discuss what you want is unlikely to be with you right through labour, so a written birth plan becomes merely a set of orders handed over to a stranger. In the words of one irritated hospital administrator: "It happens in no other branch of medicine or other professional sphere that the client imposes crucial restrictions on the professional and tells him how to do his work." The discussions you have with your caregivers and the decisions to which you come are part of the vital process of getting to know each other, so that by the time you are in labour there is an understanding which is deeper than words.

Discuss with your midwife, or the small group of midwives who will look after you, the kind of care you would like, whom you want with you during labour, what your partner's role is likely to be, how you would prefer your newborn baby to be treated, and exactly what you are hoping for with this birth. Think about interventions you would prefer to avoid, and alternative ways of coping with difficulties.

""Are you going to make a birth plan?" the midwife asked. "I think it is a good idea. We need to discuss ways in which you want to handle pain, so that I can help you. I think our ideas are much the same, but trust between us can't take the place of really knowing what you want.""

Discuss positions and movements you may want to choose, how you can get physical support for them, whether you want to use a birth pool, and your thoughts about episiotomy, the clamping and cutting of the umbilical cord, and the conduct of the third stage. Then write down your decisions about the most important issues – if possible on just one sheet of paper. Ask your caregiver how it reads, and whether she or he is happy with it. Provide one copy to go with your records, and keep another yourself. If by any chance the person you are expecting to attend you in labour is not available, this birth plan will be invaluable and give a clear idea of your preferences.

how can I arrange the room?

You and your partner will want to create your own birth space. It is a kind of "nesting". Other mammals and birds line the nest with soft hay or moss, and in most human cultures the mother and those close to her prepare a special room. The Maori birth hut was actually called "the nesting house" and traditionally, in many parts of North and South America and Asia, women built their own birth huts, often close to water so that they could bathe after the baby was born. The space for receiving the baby was always constructed to be soft and warm. The Kwakiutl of British Columbia used to dig a shallow pit and line it with soft cedar bark, and the Pima of the American South West lined their birth pits with soft rabbit skin. Making one's own birth space is an important part of human culture, which is often neglected nowadays under the assumption that this space is designed to meet the needs of the professionals who conduct the birth, rather than the mother's, and that any personal touches are introduced merely as concessions to her.

Preparing your birth space

Things you may want to get together for an out-of-hospital birth:
- Beanbags or large floor cushions.
- Camera, camcorder.
- Plenty of film, including fast film for night-time if you do not want to use a flash.
- Sanitary pads, largest size.
- Cotton pyjama tops, short nightdresses, or baggy T-shirts.
- Face cloth.
- Swimwear, so that your birth partner can go under the shower or into the bath or pool with you if you wish.
- Socks for cold feet.
- Nursing bras.
- Two small real sponges, one to suck on while the other is in a bowl of cold water.
- Small plant spray, filled with ice cold water to spray on your face.
- Cracked ice to suck.
- CDs and CD player.
- Candles, matches.

♦ Eau de cologne.

♦ Brush and comb, as well as hair-ribbons or clips to hold long hair away from your face and neck.

♦ Essential oils.

♦ Books, magazines.

♦ Snacks for birth partner and midwife.

♦ Honey, glucose drink or herb teas.

♦ Bendy straws.

♦ Rolling pin with cloth tied over it, or wooden rolling massager, for back massage.

♦ Painting, photographs, or sculpture to use as a visual focus.

♦ Champagne or other celebration drink and food for after the birth.

For birth away from home

♦ Spare can of petrol, in case your tank is empty.

♦ Coins for the phone.

♦ List of telephone numbers.

♦ Baby clothes and clothes to wear going home.

For birth at home

(Your midwife may provide some of these).

♦ Two buckets, one for sitting on, one for cleaning up.

♦ New nail brush.

♦ Bin liners.

♦ Incontinence pads for sitting on – useful if you are leaking water or if you have a heavy show, as well as for afterwards so that bedding keeps clean.

♦ Cleaning cloths.

♦ Bowl for receiving placenta.

♦ Portable lamp.

♦ Large towels, one for your use, one for your baby, and one for your midwife.

♦ Heavy plastic sheet over bed.

♦ Sheeting to protect floor.

♦ Extra heating if cold, fan if hot.

♦ Frozen peas for cold compress (wrap bag in cloth before resting against skin).

♦ Small hot-water bottle for hot compress.

♦ Birth pool or, if you want to soak in deep water and do not have a birth pool, children's modelling clay to plug the bath overflow.

What will my midwife have with her?

Delivery pack; sphygmomanometer to take blood pressure; Pinard's stethoscope and/or sonic aid; urine-testing sticks; local anaesthetic and syringes; scissors; suture material, in case of damage to the perineum; mucus extractor, in case the baby's respiratory tract needs clearing; resuscitation equipment, in case the baby needs help to breathe; intravenous set and infusion, in case of bleeding; syntometrine and syringes, in case the uterus needs help to contract to expel the placenta.

If you are going into a GP unit or birth centre, take things with you that will help to make the room your personal space, a painting, photographs, a plant, a mobile perhaps. If you are giving birth at home, you may want to choose a room that is small, dark, and private. But the birthplace does not have to be the bedroom, although a big double bed is lovely if there is room in it for the whole family just after the birth. If you have a garden, you may want to be outside for a time, and squat holding on to a tree when contractions come.

Creating comfort and the right atmosphere

When you are on dry land, have a stool or beanbag, or a bucket with a rolled towel around the rim, ready to support you in a squatting position. A lunge position with the forward knee bent is easily adopted on the stairs, or with one foot up on a small stool – or on a few encyclopedias. The banisters or bathroom towel rail may be the right height to provide a good squatting bar. In rural Africa women often kneel or squat, holding the house post that supports the roof. When my first baby was born, I spontaneously squatted grasping the heavy, bulbous legs of a Victorian table. It was a hideous table, but good and solid, and felt just right.

With your partner, think what kind of lighting would create the best atmosphere during labour and to welcome your new baby. Lamps that can be dimmed are pleasant. Would you like candles? If your birth attendant wants a bright light on your perineum to see exactly what is happening, how can this be arranged? On a bright day you may like the room flooded with sunlight, or prefer a soft glow through curtains or blinds.

"If you are tired and aching, the first thing you want to do is have a bath. That's why I have hired a birth pool."

Consider how you will warm and air the room too. You will want to be comfortably warm in labour. In winter you may like to give birth on a hearthrug or a couch in front of the flickering flames of a guarded open fire, or in summer in a room opening on to the garden. You may feel very hot in the second stage and want to have a window wide open or an electric fan available. The baby is emerging from a hot-house atmosphere inside your body, and needs to be born into warm air, so a fan heater that can be switched on as the birth approaches is a good idea.

Using sounds Think together about the things around you that you will find comforting during labour, and that will enhance your positive visualization of what is happening in your body. If you would like to have some background music playing, plan this together. Practise your relaxation techniques whilst playing this music, so that you associate it with complete release of mind and body. The sounds you choose don't have to be music. You could record the dawn chorus, or waves breaking on the shore. One of my babies was born as a blackbird sang in the apple tree outside my bedroom window. It was an enormously reassuring, happy sound, and I felt that nature was conspiring with me to make the birth beautiful for all of us.

Aromatherapy and smells For good smells there is a wide range of aromatherapy oils to choose. A study of aromatherapy in more than 8,000 births suggests that clary sage and camomile reduce pain, lavender and frankincense treat anxiety and fear, and peppermint is effective against nausea and vomiting.* Be warned that clary sage smells like wet dog! You need to have a head cold or be very fond of dogs! Rose oil is delicious, but expensive, the reason why it could not be tested at the Oxford Radcliffe Maternity Hospital. Midwife Ethel Burns introduced aromatherapy there in 1990. One of her aims was to cut the rate of women receiving opiates for pain relief, since pethidine, the most widely used drug, is a very poor analgesic and has side effects for both mother and baby. This hospital has the lowest rate of pethidine of all major maternity hospitals in Britain. Aromatherapy changes the whole atmosphere of the birth room. It is not only the mother who becomes more relaxed. The people helping her often feel calmer and happier, too. You may like to have scented candles, bunches of lavender, or flowers in the room. When my fourth baby was born, my bedroom was full of bowls of hyacinths, and I always associate the heady scent of hyacinths with that particular birth.

images of birth

An important part of your preparation for birth is nothing to do with exercises or information: it is simply to daydream.

When you relax and focus on positive sensory images of birth, you open up possibilities for a richer and deeper experience. These images should always be realistic in the sense that they are based on acknowledgement that labour is stressful, the power of the uterus is awesome, when the cervix is opening to its full extent it is usually painful, and that when the baby's head is in your vagina there is an incredible sensation of pressure. You can anticipate and acknowledge all these sensations in a positive way.

The power of words

The words you use are vital elements in these anticipatory fantasies. Language is never neutral. It presents a view of the world. Most words we have about pregnancy and birth are not only man-made but also medical. A woman is an "elderly primigravida" or "high risk". She has "an untried pelvis". Doctors' names are attached to processes in women's bodies as if these medical men had somehow invented them. The contractions in late pregnancy are known as "Braxton-Hicks". Dilatation of the cervix must follow the "Friedman curve". To use medical language is to impose on yourself a medical view of birth. Sometimes medical terms are the only words available, so we need to translate them into women's language, and create words that have immediate meaning for us in terms of our own feelings and the ways in which we can express ourselves through our bodies.

Body images

Your pelvis, for example, is not just an anatomical structure, a piece of architecture through which the fetus is pushed. When you rock your pelvis with your baby nestled inside, it is like a cradle. As you sing, hum, or chant, it becomes a resonator. Sometimes it may feel like a mysterious cave, or a treasure chest that holds the power of the uterus. In a woman's pelvis the ebb and flow of menstrual tides take place and, when the time is right, the drama of birth is enacted. You can create your own images. You need not use second-hand ones. These anticipatory fantasies derived from sensory experience need not all be visual. They can be auditory, for example, based on passages from music and ideas of cadence, harmony, rhythm, and being in tune with your body.

As you reach out to touch your newborn, you realize that you are already familiar with that firm, round head, the pointed bottom, and those sturdy little legs.

They can be tactile too. A feeling of the baby moving inside you is one of intense and often surprising touch. As the uterus contracts and your baby moves down to enter the world, you feel intense pressure, your waters may break with a soft splash, and you are aware of your baby's firm head sliding down – solid and rounded as a grapefruit – and of quivering, throbbing heat as the head crowns. As it slips forwards and you reach down to feel it, your fingers touch soft, wet hair, and you are astonished at the otherness of this little creature who has for so long been a part of yourself but is now being born from your body.

Kinetic images may come to mind too. Your breathing dances, you get into the swing of contractions, swimming over each as it rises in crescendo, or breasting it like a great ocean wave. You float, you ride, you ski down the mountain slopes, you leap into the void. I shall never forget an Israeli woman who, as each contraction swelled up, proclaimed: "Gates of Jerusalem, open for me!" And for her this was the intense image that most accurately expressed the sense of her body opening wide as she gave birth.

The imagery that is likely to be helpful to you during labour will include active verbs of opening, releasing, spreading, unfolding, and fanning out.

As contractions sweep through you, concepts that suggest power, energy, strength, and, perhaps, storm and even whirlwind suddenly make sense, along with wave and water fantasies – verbs such as stream, pool, flood, gush, flow and cascade. And all over the world, in many different cultures, women use visual images of fruit ripening and of the baby's head like a hard bud in the centre of a flower's unfurling petals.

As you read about childbirth, and whenever you take time to relax and enjoy your anticipatory fantasies, create your own images and dreams that will give positive meaning to all the sensations of labour. Doing this will help you to savour fully an adventure that can be among the most thrilling, intense and satisfying experiences of your life.

Is water birth safe?

Q A Where shall we set up the pool?

The ideal room for a birth pool is probably on the ground floor, with one door opening out onto a garden and another onto a darkened, comfortable room where you can escape the pressures of the outside world and sink deeply into your own sensations.

If it is warm weather, you can then labour part of the time in the fresh air, and withdraw to your womb-like room or float peacefully in the pool the rest of the time.

The important thing is to be free to move between these different environments and not feel committed to water birth, come what may.

Q A Are the floor boards strong enough?

If you want to have the pool in an upstairs room and the floor is wooden, check with the people from whom you are hiring it or a friendly builder that the floor can take its weight when it is filled with water. This will be about one tonne.

Q A Can the hose-pipe reach the taps?

There are two hoses with the pool. One has attachments to connect it securely to the taps. Allow a good hour to fill the pool. The second enables you to run off water, so that you can feed in fresh hot water through the other hose or empty the pool. To avoid having hosepipes snaking all over the place, the pool is best located not far from a sink or bath.

*Can the pool be emptied easily? Think about where the waste water will run – perhaps straight into a drain or garden. A pool equipped with an electric pump can be emptied rapidly.

Q A How do we heat the water?

It helps to have an efficient domestic hot water supply. If necessary, turn up the thermostat on the immersion heater, but be very careful if you have other children in the house. Some pools have heaters similar to those used in aquaria. Although they maintain the water at a comfortable temperature, they are not powerful enough to

heat it from cold, and you may not like the idea of having a heater in the pool when you are in it. The pool should have a plastic cover that, even without a heater, retains heat well, so that once filled the pool will stay warm for eight to ten hours.

Q A What temperature should the water be?

Around blood temperature is right. Really hot water is not good for the baby, who while inside you is hotter than you. The air around the pool should be warm so that after the birth the baby does not lose heat rapidly and you can cuddle her while still sitting in the water. In the second stage you may get very hot, and it feels good if the water is cool. This helps you mobilize your energy to push the baby out and stimulates the urge to bear down.

Q A When should we get the pool?

Set the pool up about ten days before the baby is due and use it for relaxation and centering down into positive thoughts about birth. It helps to alleviate late-pregnancy backache, and feels good if you have clusters of painful Braxton-Hicks contractions or a long lead into labour.

Q How can the water be kept clean?

Empty the pool every 24 hours or so, and refill with clean water. It is usually not difficult to keep the water clean. A plastic sieve can be used to scoop any debris out of the water.

Q Is it safe to leave the baby underwater after the birth?

No. At birth, gently lift your baby's head free of the water. Don't jerk it up suddenly. This may cause a short cord to beak. Though it is not an emergency, and a midwife knows what to do, it is best avoided, and the cord can be left intact to stop pulsating by itself.

Being in water eases pain, and enables you to move more freely and to explore positions in which your pelvis is at its widest, such as wide-open kneeling.

Water birth

You may want to use water – with the bath, shower, jacuzzi, or a special birth pool. (There are details of where to hire a pool on page 192.) If so, do you want your partner to be in the water with you or not? You may feel differently when you are in labour, but plan ahead for a range of possibilities and experiment with different positions and movements in water.

Of course you are concerned about safety. A paediatric study of over 4,000 births in water in the UK between 1994 and 1996 compared with more conventional births to women not at any special risk, shows that water birth is not dangerous. It is as safe for the baby to be born in water as in air.*

your birth partner

Sharing the experience of childbirth with someone who is close to you helps give you strength and confidence. When you have a baby at home this person is usually your sexual partner because birth occurs quite naturally as a part of the flow of your relationship. When birth is in a GP unit or birth centre, you may want your sexual partner with you as this special person, or perhaps you want someone else – a friend or relative.

male anxieties about birth

In the past, men distanced themselves from birth, both its physiological and emotional aspects. It was not "manly" to do anything else. They strode the hospital corridors while their wives laboured. They crouched smoking in the fathers' waiting room. They went to a pub and drank themselves silly to anaesthetize their fears. Or they tried to concentrate on work as if nothing important was happening. They denied the strength of their own anxiety. It was as if a script was already written for them and they had to accept their allotted roles. Men lost out as well as women. The taboo on tenderness, of which this was one example, meant that they were expected to be strong to shoulder burdens, to earn money to support their wives and children, and to protect territory, but were not allowed to be aware of the intricacies of human emotion or the subtleties of relationships. If they were in touch with their feelings, they had to put on an act and pretend that they were tough and strong. The role stereotype was basically ape-like, not human.

In the span of 30 years, fathers' involvement in childbirth in Western culture, novel in the 60s, has come to be accepted as

"Chris was looking at the baby with his complete attention, his face transfigured with happiness and wonder. He looked like a small child seeing something more wonderful than he had ever seen before."

normal. Maybe the idea of fathers at birth contained the seed of "the new man" – the male personality who is not grabbing, fighting, and crude, but who can be nurturing and tender. But, in spite of many fathers now attending the births of their babies, this new man is a much heralded but still rare creature – a new and endangered species in a rough, tough world. Yet each time a woman gives birth and a man has the opportunity to share the experience and to grow in understanding, there is at least a chance that not only a baby but a man with a deeper awareness and sensitivity will be born.

On the other hand it is easy to be over-optimistic about the changes that can be brought about when fathers are involved in childbirth in hospital. A concerned, caring father can help with communication and give his partner strong emotional support. But hospitals are organized so that even the most determined man may go along with the system all too easily and fail to give the support a woman needs.

"We felt strongly that our child should emerge into her father's arms and share that first breath of life in the intimate bond of the family."

When fathers began to be at births back in the 60s, their presence was at first resisted by many doctors and midwives, who felt that their territory was threatened. But within a few years fathers came to be warmly welcomed, as staff realized that most of them turned into subordinate, well-behaved members of the birth "team", who could be relied upon to help control the woman's behaviour, keep her calm, and make her "see reason" when staff wished to intervene in the labour against her wishes.*

Men still often feel out of place in hospital childbirth, and do everything they can to maintain good relations with staff, to be polite and compliant, and to prevent the woman "making a fuss" or drawing attention to herself. They go into hospital with the firm purpose of giving labour support, but many are cowed into submission by the whole atmosphere of the unit and by the evident authority of the senior men who are in charge. Fathers often feel violent emotions welling up inside them

"Nicholas was where I needed him about ten seconds before I knew where that was! I felt supported, but not pushed, by all three of them."

because of how their partners are being treated, yet are conditioned by their education to block the expression of disturbing feelings, and to be obedient team members. In this state of mind they are inclined to play the hospital game, to collude with the medical system, and women are left feeling isolated and abandoned.

Most obstetricians are men, and it is unlikely that this has occurred by chance. They want to control women in the most essentially female activity of giving birth. So they invent machinery to enable them to do this more effectively. It is almost a truism to say that men like machines, enjoy tinkering with them, and rely on them more than women. It is only a truism, because it is usually women who operate and understand the idiosyncrasies of electric irons and kettles, vacuum cleaners, washing machines, dishwashers, mixers, sewing machines, typewriters, and wordprocessors. Because men are accustomed to being in control of women, obstetricians manage childbirth – or at least achieve a semblance of management – with electronic equipment. Prospective fathers are often reassured when they see the technology available in the modern hospital, whereas their female partners tend to be disturbed by it. Of course there are some men who are made equally anxious by all this high-tech gear, just as there are women who breathe a sigh of relief and believe that nothing can go wrong if it is to hand. But they are probably in the minority.

> "Philip fixed me with his eyes gently and kindly, yet insistently. He never allowed me to sink into the pain. Eye contact and simultaneous breathing with him got me through the contractions."

Fathers' sharing in the birth experience can be the stimulus for men's freedom to nurture, and a sign of changing relationships between men and women. In the same way, women's freedom to give birth at home is a political decision, an assertion of our determination to reclaim the experience of birth. Birth at home is about changing society.

A father:
> "The birth was made much easier by being in comfortable, familiar and planned surroundings, and having midwives who were our friends, rather than the staff of an institution, visiting our own home and helping us through a difficult but exciting and joyful time."

The deeper meanings of birth

Sharing the experience of birth can be a peak event in a loving relationship, something that is never forgotten. Rahima Baldwin, who helps run a birth centre where half the parents are Arab, speaks movingly of "the profound moment when the father whispers the al-adhan, or call to prayer," to his newbom child. Men who were not at all sure at first that they wanted to be present, say afterwards: "I wouldn't have missed it for the world." For many it is as if suddenly they are face to face with life's real meaning, and a power even more overwhelming than sexual desire.

When women are asked afterwards what their partners did that helped, they often say: "It was just that he was there." Being present in the moment, not distracting or distracted, but right there with her, is the essence of being a birth partner. It is nothing to do with coaching the woman, as the father's role is often described in North American childbirth "'education'". It is not a matter of complicated techniques, but of giving her complete and focused concentration.

It is possible to be physically present with a woman in labour and not be there at all. I remember accompanying one couple having a hospital birth for whom the event was a truce in a long-drawn-out battle. The husband, who was a doctor, brought his transistor radio into the delivery room and, as his wife was pushing the baby out, he switched on the news and listened to it intently, until I suggested that this was the wrong time and place for it and asked him to get behind her to support her head and shoulders.

It may be that hospital delivery rooms and women in the second stage of labour were so commonplace for him that he did not see any need to be emotionally involved. Or he may have been trying to punish his wife. Or perhaps he was trying to protect himself from overwhelming emotion, and was frightened that he might feel too much.

Preparing together

Your birth partner should prepare with you for the birth, not just be called in when you start labour. He or she should be someone who understands your needs and knows exactly when it is appropriate to give help and when to stand back.

Men are often poorly prepared for the experience of childbirth. A study of what fathers actually did when they had planned to act as "labour coaches" in a Canadian hospital revealed that they spent a lot of time trying to hide their feelings and worrying that they were not being useful.*

Though most had attended childbirth classes, when it came to labour itself they were not able to help in the way they had expected, and their emotions proved very different from those anticipated. The hospital environment often inhibits a birth partner from giving a woman full support and puts him under great stress. He feels surrounded by experts, is scared of doing the wrong thing and, if the woman becomes distressed as labour progresses, he becomes increasingly anxious. Birth in an out-of-hospital setting provides an environment in which the birth partner can also be himself. He doesn't feel that he has to put on an act.

feelings about birth

Anyone who is present at a birth brings to it their own emotions, their own expectations, their fear and hope, and their love. As a baby is born, there is not only the mother's birth passion, but the often intense emotions of all others involved. This is why emotional preparation is vital. Childbirth education is not just a matter of learning what happens and knowing how to help. It should be a process that leads to greater self-awareness.

Whether your birth partner is your sexual partner or some other person with whom you have chosen to share the experience, it is important to talk together about your feelings beforehand.

◆ What is most important to you about the birth?
◆ What do you want of your birth partner?
◆ How does your birth partner feel about this?
◆ What kind of help will your partner need to give?
◆ How does your partner feel about this?

Emotions about birth are often complex and powerful. You can explore feelings further by each going on to finish the statement, "When I think about the birth, I feel . . ." Listen to each other without judgement and, if some of these emotions turn out to be threatening to the other person, do not try to change them or protest that there is no need to feel like this. Just accept them.

Can you remember your first contact with birth as a child? As I talk with couples, I find that earliest memories are often negative. Adults may recall bewilderment when their mother was whisked off to hospital, they were left without her, and then presented with a baby who replaced them. They may also remember hushed, pitying voices as "female problems" were discussed, or an aunt's "bad time" as women talked in shocked whispers about the number of stitches she had. All these experiences colour

"When I was in transition, I said 'I'm bloody well not doing this again,' and he reminded me: 'You must be nearly fully dilated. It won't be long now! Take one contraction at a time.' When I did that, the pain was suddenly manageable."

our view of birth as adults, even if they only serve to make us determined to do things differently for ourselves.

Many men are not sure that they can handle seeing the woman they love in pain, or cope with being so close to the sheer physicality of birth. If you have seen a birth film together, talk about your feelings as you watched it as well. Viewing a birth film is very different from actually being fully involved in a birth. With a film you are merely a spectator, and there is nothing you can do about it. In a birth you are needed and caught up in the yearning and excitement of the moment. It is the difference between watching a film of surfers on Bondi Beach and actually being there and riding the waves yourself.

Talking about how your partner has felt in the past when you have been in pain, or were ill or especially vulnerable, can also help to deepen your understanding of each other. What did you want from your partner then? The pain of birth is functional, creative, positive. It is pain with a purpose. When a woman feels trapped and unable to control what other people do to her pain is turned into *suffering*.

In an intimate atmosphere the physicality of birth can be close to that of love-making. The swelling uterus straining against the abdominal wall, the woman's quickened breathing, her damp skin and hair and shining eyes, the astonishing urge to push, and the energy that pours through her, the grunts and moans as she presses the baby down, the bulging perineum, the top of the baby's head like a wrinkled walnut in her vagina, and then oozing through – all these elements in birth are sexual when they are not made medical in the context of hospital care.

Sharing birth dreams

Women often dream more during pregnancy. Dreams that were previously grey turn technicoloured. Men may dream too, and their dreams may express hopes and anxieties about birth. Sometimes there is fear of losing the woman, of the baby being abnormal, or of not being able to measure up to what is required of them. While I am not suggesting that you go into lengthy dream analysis, dreams can often provide clues to the problems we are trying to sort out in our lives and the challenges we face. It helps just to realize this and to say, "Yes, I am worried about it," and to think whether there is some positive action that you can take to deal with the challenge.

Even when there is nothing practical to be done, a simple acknowledgement of the fear often enables you to handle it.

is it a good idea to have a woman friend to help me?

Sometimes a man wants to be present at the birth of his child but feels that he cannot take entire responsibility for giving emotional support. If this is the case then having another person present as well, a woman who understands birth, may be a good idea. This person may be called a "doula", a Greek word meaning "the woman who serves" and in France, a "monitrice", which means "the woman who watches and is aware". When a couple are together, the task for the doula is not to take over, but to support them both. As one doula put it: "I am there to help a woman, just like her mother or father was when she learned to ride a bicycle. During birth I am like the parent who held on to the back of the bicycle until the rider had some experience and felt safe and turned around to see that she had been riding on her own for quite some time."*

Choosing the right partners

The notion that a woman can have only one companion with her during labour, and that this person must be the baby's father, stems from the time in the late 60s when fathers were first allowed in delivery rooms, and women were told that no one else could possibly come because there was no room. Over and over again, senior midwives and doctors explained to couples "there just isn't space". Notices were often put up by delivery suite doors: "No admission. Fathers only." This was hard on single mothers and on any woman who wanted a woman friend with her during labour instead of a man.

Now in many countries the father's presence is unquestioned. But in ritualizing the attendance of fathers and making it almost mandatory, women are denied the right to choose another person, or perhaps several people with different qualities to offer. It is only in a home setting that these decisions can be made freely; and it is important that they are made, and that a reluctant or anxious father does not hang around simply because he lives there and everyone assumes that he is the obvious birth partner.

what does a birth partner do?

You are for the woman you are supporting an anchor in a stormy sea. Being able to remain calmly confident during the labour is the single most important quality needed from a birth partner.

There are many ways of giving comfort when the going gets tough and of refreshing her if she feels so tired that she wishes it was all over. You will learn about these skills in childbirth classes and have a chance to rehearse them and find out which are likely to suit her best. When you do this in a group with other couples, you can learn a great deal from each other and can also share ideas.

"I didn't need him to do anything. I didn't want to be told what to do. Being able to rely on him, knowing he wouldn't leave me, seeing him there smiling as I came out of every contraction, that was what I needed."

It often helps to use words and phrases that were used in the childbirth classes – those that held most meaning for you. They can be very simple, such as "open", "release", "lovely", or "good", or repeated phrases, such as "let it flow", "you are strong", "you are doing really well", "that's another one gone", or "we're getting there". I have found myself in the role of birth partner in countries where I have been studying women's experiences of birth and have not spoken the language. All I needed to do was know a few words, such as "softly", "breathe", "gently", "open wide" and "beautiful", with which to reach out to a woman, and these have been enough to give strong birth support. I aim to be beside a woman, not over her but with her. Separated by culture, education, and language, we yet encounter each other as sisters.

No woman wants to be hectored or cajoled whilst in labour. If help is offered without empathy, it can seem as if the other person is taking over, and a woman may think: "Who's having this baby, you or me?" So keep words to the minimum.

"It was good having him to squeeze tight, and I knew he wouldn't mind how hard I squeezed. With anyone else I would have felt bound to apologize, but I just clung on to him."

Whatever techniques birth partners acquire, however much they learn, the essence of what they give to the woman in birth is that they are her lovers and friends, not assistants to the midwife, barefoot doctors, or labour "coaches".

A birth partner should be sensitively aware of what a woman needs at any given moment.

touch, massage and holding

When a woman feels tossed and lost and broken by fierce contractions coming in quick succession, being held firmly helps her feel safe. Your hand stroking lightly or massaging her deeply can relieve pain even when it is very threatening, depending on where and how the touch is given. Any kind of physical contact from a person whom she trusts can, if given with discretion and sensitivity, help her relax in a situation which is stressful. One strong benefit of not being in an alien environment during the labour is that you are much less likely to feel inhibited in giving her your physical support and caring for her freely through touch.

During pregnancy you can explore together ways of touching and holding, so that just a look or gesture from her will indicate to you when and where she wants to feel the reassurance and energy that is given by a loved hand.

Before you practise, prepare some massage oil – vegetable oil or nut oil lightly scented with any essential oil that she finds relaxing. Then she strips down to her underclothes and settles in a warm, comfortable place, well supported by pillows.

Stroking

You can make contact with the baby by stroking the mother's abdomen lightly. You will notice that this touch needs to be made with really relaxed, warm hands, so it is worth spending a few minutes loosening hands before starting by shaking them vigorously from the wrists as if flicking water from the finger-tips. For all massage, your shoulders need to be loose too. If they are tight, tension is conveyed down the arm into the hand and can even cause pain.

When contractions are coming every two or three minutes a woman often feels that she needs an anchor in the stormy sea of labour, and wants to be upright and firmly held.

Slow, light stroking over the lower abdomen can feel good in labour, especially before 5 cm dilatation of the cervix. If you are slightly to one side of her, an oiled hand can be drawn from underneath the far curve of her abdomen in an arc down over the place where her cervix is dilating, and then up again over the nearer side, followed by the other hand using a similar smooth movement in the same direction. The resulting light finger-tip massage seems to be stroking the baby's head.

Shoulder massage

The tension that results in over-breathing and hyperventilation starts in the shoulders, and a shoulder massage helps her loosen these muscles. You are behind her, fingers resting on her shoulders, and massage firmly with thumbs in the valleys either side of her spine. Then try moving the thumbs slowly and firmly in a circular motion over her shoulder blades.

Back massage

Long, slow, sweeping movements with the hands down either side of her spine can help her relax completely between contractions, so that she does not carry over tension from one contraction to another. First the hands rest on the shoulders. Then one hand is moved firmly,

The role of the birth partner

"lovely", or "good", or repeated phrases, such as "let it flow", "you are strong", "you are doing really well", "that's another one gone", or "we're getting there".

Q&A I've heard that a partner should "coach" a woman in labour. Is this what I ought to do?

No one wants to be hectored or cajoled in labour. If help is offered without empathy, it can seem as if the other person is taking over, and a woman may think: "Who's having this baby, you or me?" So keep words to the minimum.

Q&A Should a birth partner attend childbirth classes?

Yes. In classes you learn ways of getting "in tune" with contractions and conserving energy, have a chance to rehearse them and find out which are likely to suit you best. When you do this in a group with other couples, you learn a great deal from each other and can share ideas.

Q&A What sort of encouragement can I give?

It often helps to use words that were used in the classes – those that held most meaning for you both. They can be very simple, such as "open", "release",

Q&A What is the most important thing I can do to help?

For the woman you are supporting you are her anchor in a stormy sea. Being able to remain calmly confident is the single most important quality needed. Whatever techniques birth partners learn – massage and offering strong physical support so that she can move around, for example – the essence of what they give the woman is that they are her lovers and friends, not assistants to the midwife, barefoot doctors, or "coaches".

Offering support and assistance during labour

In the peace between contractions you may like to use some of the following phrases or questions so that the mother can be your guide:

♦ Do you want to be touched, or not?

♦ Would you like me to move my hands, or keep them still?

♦ Will you guide my hands?

♦ Heavier? Lighter?

♦ Shall I talk you through the next contraction, or be quiet?

♦ Show me how to hold you.

♦ Does it help if I breathe with you?

Don't say these things all at once, use your words with discretion. The woman in labour leads. You follow.

without haste, sweeping down her back. When this hand reaches her bottom, the other hand joins in the movement, and slowly sweeps down the other side, as the first hand is replaced on her shoulder, and so on. You will need to have a relaxed body to do this easily, as this massage is only satisfying when you literally get into the rhythmic swing of it.

When there is back pain, it is usually most concentrated at the sacrum, the big bone where her pelvis is attached to your spine, or to one side of this. Pain in this region is helped by very firm circular massage from the heel of the palm with the other hand resting over it, so that pressure comes from the weight of your back down the shoulders and arms into the hands. When you practise this, try the effect of being at different angles to her body, because the pressure she feels will be different depending on whether it is exerted in an upward or downward direction. It may be most effective when you are near her shoulders, so that this pressure is exerted downwards on your sacro-lumbar ligaments.

Foot massage

You hold her feet in your lap and squeeze her foot above and below her calf muscles front and back, and then massage the soles of her feet with your thumbs. This can be done between strong contractions. As the next contraction builds up, your hands are stilled, and firm thumb pressure is exerted just below the big toe of each foot, slightly in to the next toe. If you experiment with this massage, you will find a spot on the foot in which strong pressure produces a slight buzzing sensation. It is an acupressure (shiatsu) point which will help to prevent pain.

"My midwife was warm, loving, and calm. She massaged my feet and kept encouraging me. I looked into Nick's eyes and saw the love he has for me. This kept me going through a 36-hour labour."

Giving counter-pressure

She may appreciate firm counter-pressure rather than moving touch. So much is happening inside her during labour that any movement may be distracting and break her concentration. Counter-pressure is particularly effective for relieving low back pain if strong hands rest one on top of the other over exactly the right spot on the back, and your weight is allowed to flow down your arms as you press. As the baby presses lower, she may like this pressure over her buttocks.

Kneading

Deep massage into the flesh and underlying muscles can help her cope with sensations which might otherwise seem preposterous and threatening. As the baby's head presses against her rectum and anus, it may feel as if she is about to empty her bowels. Then, as the head fans out all the tissues, it feels like a huge ball just behind her anus. To help her relax her buttock and pelvic floor muscles, you can knead her buttocks using thumbs or thumbs and fingers as if kneading bread dough.

Holding

Holding is helpful not only for physical support in upright positions, but when she just needs to know that someone is there, focused entirely on her, or when she wants to be steadied and anchored.

Some good holding positions with which you can experiment are: supporting the back of her shoulders; encircling a wrist; grasping her feet; holding the bony ridge of her pelvis on either side; and cradling her head with a hand on each side or one hand cupped over the back of her head. You should stay quite still, feeling and sharing the power that is sweeping through her body.

You can find much more about touch, massage, and holding in my book *Pregnancy and Childbirth*, details of which are on page 193

moving around

When a woman is in labour, it will help if she has already explored with her movements and positions she is most likely to find comfortable, bearing in mind as she does that upright positions will enable her uterus to contract freely and the baby's head to rotate and descend. One great advantage of home birth is that you both already know exactly what you can use for comfort and physical support – walls, window ledges, and furniture – and you don't have to use any special apparatus such as a squatting bar or birth chair.

You can experiment with the following labour movements and positions together before the birth:

♦ She walks about and then, as she imagines a contraction, leans forward on to you with her legs well apart and knees unlocked. She can try this facing you, behind you, and at your side. Experiment with you standing with your back against the wall for support. Then try it sitting on a chair or table.

♦ Find out in which of these positions that you have just practised you can rub her back easily. She walks around again, and this time imagines contractions coming with low backache. You massage her firmly in the small of her back where her pelvis joins her spine. Massage is best done at one side or both sides of the spine, not right on it, and using the heel of the palm rather than the fingers or flat of the hand.

♦ She walks again and when an imaginary contraction starts, leans flat forward on to a wall in any way that is comfortable. Massage her as she stands in this position.

♦ She sits facing the back of an upright chair, leaning over a pillow on the back of the chair, with her shoulders rounded, feet flat on the floor. You can massage her back in this position.

♦ Now she turns so that she sits on the chair in the conventional way. Kneel in front of her and she can lean over you.

There are many other positions and movements you can explore, using you for support or being massaged by you, or sometimes both at once. Other positions to try are:

♦ Kneeling with legs wide apart, leaning forwards with her head on a pillow on a chair in front of her;

♦ Kneeling upright;

♦ Half-kneeling, half-squatting, with one foot flat on the floor;

♦ An all-fours position; and squatting, leaning forwards with your hands on the floor.

In many of these positions she may also welcome additional physical support from you.

Once she feels confident being supported by you in a range of positions, explore movements she may want to make. With some of these she may like you to be still. With others it feels best if you move with her in the same rhythm.

♦ She rocks her pelvis on all fours while you rest a hand at either side of her pelvis.

♦ She squats, leaning forwards and holding on to you, and then rocks her pelvis to and fro.

♦ She kneels and leans over you, while you are on all fours in front of her, and rocks her pelvis in this position.

When the second stage of labour starts and she is pushing the baby out, she doesn't have to go to bed unless she wants to. She may have the ideal bed – a four-poster – and be able to squat holding on to one of the posts, or a bed with a solid headboard which she can grasp as she kneels facing it. If she is using a bed, it is best if the mattress is firm. But it may feel better to be on a clean sheet on the floor. Explore some of the positions she may want to use:

♦ She stands with you behind her holding her elbows, wrists, or hands, whichever is most comfortable. If you are taller than her, you should keep a straight back, bending your knees slightly.

♦ She stands in front of and facing you, with her hands clasped around your neck.

♦ With you sitting behind her, she sits upright between your legs, with her knees drawn up and legs well apart. Use pillows as necessary for extra support for you both.

With all your preparations together, however, you will need to be flexible so that she can do whatever feels right at the time of birth, even if it is not what she planned. It is important for you to know when to be silent, when to give her her own space, when not to intrude and when to let her flow with the labour.

The power of birth is like the strength of water cascading in a mighty rush down the hillside. It is the power of seas and tides, the power of mountains moving. There is no way of ignoring it. She cannot fight it. No amount of technique can enable her to be in control of it as she might be in control of a car or a computer. You should aim not to manage, conduct, or coach her through this experience, but rather to give her strength and confidence as she allows her body to open and your baby to press through it to life.

sharing the experience

Having a strong support group, sharing the experience of pregnancy, swapping your accounts of interviews with obstetricians, of hospital visits, of previous labours and dealing with the medical system, can help you discover what your rights are and learn effective strategies. During labour, too, you may want to have close friends or family with you. They can increase your confidence and give a great deal of comfort.

the need for support

When you plan a birth outside hospital, it helps to have a network of supporters – other couples and women – with whom you can share experiences, develop effective strategies for coping and work together towards change. You will probably find other like-minded people in your antenatal class, among your midwife's other clients and in childbirth organizations (see those listed on page 196). If you are having a baby in a birth centre, you will be able to talk to newly delivered women and their partners over a cup of tea in the kitchen when you visit, and will soon find that you are part of a group of prospective and new parents who support the birth centre. In the same way the groups formed to defend GP units that are threatened with closure, in countries where the policy is one of centralization, are strongly cohesive and militant in a very positive, celebratory way, and you will make new friends and discover many others who think the same way as you do.

In most countries a woman who wants a home birth tends to be isolated, has to fight a lonely battle, and may be treated by doctors as if she is suffering from severe emotional problems. Sometimes a hospital obstetrician has gone so far as to threaten a woman with psychiatric detention or with having her newborn baby confiscated because of her "irresponsibility". It is too much to expect a woman to be able to handle this hostility alone. In her book, *Midwives and Medical Men*, Jean Donnison says of women seeking home birth that they need "the patience of Job, the courage of Joan of Arc, and the political skill of a Metternich".*

Support from other women

Traditionally a woman in childbirth has always had other women helping her. As well as the midwife, there were friends, family members and neighbours who gave emotional and practical support during and after the birth. In 1658, Ralph Josselin recorded in his diary that his wife's labour had been so quick that, besides the midwife and nurse (for the baby), "only two or three women more got to her but God supplied all, young Mrs Harlakenden got up to us very speedily, and some others".*

Other women still give support to women in childbirth in most Third World countries. When anthropologists are present at a birth, it is often quite difficult for them to find out who exactly the midwife is, because she is one of a group of women helpers engaged in a task within a non-medical context. Childbirth is like bread-baking, laundering, or cheese-making-activities that involve a community of women working together. In our own past, and cross-culturally, every adult woman was expected to know what to do in childbirth and how to help other women. She might have a recipe for a strengthening broth to be taken during labour, know which herbs could be used to stimulate the uterus, or have a lodestone or charm to help the birth go well.

"We were sure that we didn't want to have our child come into a group of strangers, but rather into the loving circle of family and friends in a familiar setting."

Throughout Europe in medieval times, when a woman started labour, she called on other women in the neighbourhood, who came bringing food to sustain them all during the the labour and for celebration after the birth, and plenty of strong drink. Men were turned out of the house as women took over. These women would later testify at the baptism of the child, and were referred to as God sibs, which literally means "sisters in God". Men must have resented this female takeover, and in English the words "God sib" gradually became changed in male usage to "gossip".

In pioneer times in North America women relied heavily on what was known in Canada as "turn-about" help. It carried on the old European tradition but with a new urgency, since many of them were in isolated communities. Women had to be able to heal illness, mend bones, comfort the dying, and help one another in childbirth. When a baby was on the way, they made each other baby clothes and sewed beautiful bed quilts and then, when labour started, cooked meals, did the housework, took over the woman's other duties, such as milking the cows, and cared for the mother and her family for some days after the birth, until she was fit to take up again the heavy work that was an integral part of life on a pioneer farm.*

These women often travelled some distance between their own homes, where they had work of their own to do, and the new mother's home. And, if a woman went into labour when the helper was in the middle of a major domestic project, the helper brought her own work along:

I recall one time a man coming 18 miles in a sleigh to take my grandmother to his wife who was expecting a baby. My grandmother had mixed bread dough earlier in the day, so she packed the pan of dough in with her in this sleigh, which was comfortably warm with lots of blankets and quilts and heated stones. When she arrived at the farmer's home, the dough had risen enough to bake, so she baked it in the stove in his kitchen and, after she delivered the baby, the husband drove my grandmother back home with all her bread baked.

There was rarely any exchange of money for this kind of "turn-about" help. Families repaid each other with gifts of produce, assistance with farm work, or with building and equipping a house. The strong links forged between women at times of great significance in their lives formed a basis for the new communities that were being created.

"It mattered to me that the women there had had babies themselves and knew what it was like. They weren't shocked or surprised by anything. They stayed calm, down-to-earth, and always comforting."

Postnatal support was given as a matter of course too, and women sent over cooked meals for the new mother and her family. As one midwife in an isolated fishing community in Newfoundland put it, "There was always other women from around coming and looking out to things that needed to be done. No one starved, let me tell you, when a woman was lyin' in."* In this community it was

Birth has always drawn women to reach out and help each other and to welcome a new life.

the custom on the last day of lying in to have an "upsitting day", when the neighbouring women, together with the midwife, gathered in the new mother's house for tea and "Groaning Cake", which was often baked by the father.*

In the past no woman had to labour alone or among strangers, and no mother lacked postnatal nurture. Isolation and loneliness came with the move from home to hospital. Even in hospital, having another woman there who is responsible to you, not to the hospital, and who has no medical function, may bring a great deal of comfort, ease labour and result in a better outcome. When research was done in Guatemala comparing the labours of women going into hospital with no support from other women with those of others who had one-to-one support from a caring woman, even one they did not know before, the results were spectacularly in favour of the woman-to-woman support.* A Canadian study found that those women who had their partners with them and had also been assigned a "monitrice" were admitted to hospital later in labour, were more likely to require no medication during childbirth, and to have an intact perineum.*

With home birth the presence of other women in the family and female friends occurs quite spontaneously without the need to obtain permission or worry about protocol. In such a setting women rediscover an ancient role in childbirth and the postpartum weeks, and can form a strong, loving group to nurture the mother and be in company with her through a significant life transition.

"I'd never had that feeling so strongly before, of women sharing a process they understood and in complete harmony with each other, it was like a dance in which you all hear the same music and move accordingly, without having to talk about it."

Doctors often find the presence of other women during a birth very threatening to their professional status. Hospital nurses and midwives may feel uneasy in the same way. They fear that they will lose control of the patient. So in a hospital you may be told that there is "no room", or that they might "get in the way" or distract you and make the labour go badly.

giving the right kind of help

It is undoubtedly true that a lively party going on around you during labour may prove irritating, and contradictory advice or general chat can be as intrusive, in its own way, as obstetric intervention. Any women who are with you should be able to tune in to how you are feeling and what you want of them. Michel Odent believes that the presence of other people at the birth, even the partner, may prevent a woman from trusting her instincts and from "being on another planet", as he calls the state of focused inward concentration when labour is at its height.

But when women are bonded together in a task – whether in a workplace outside the home, a kitchen, or a birth room – there is a special quality about the work they do. There is a common give-and-take in their interaction, an understanding that develops between them – often with no need for words – that can be described only by the word "sisterhood". I am not claiming that something similar cannot exist for men too – only that childbirth is a female task, and that women sharing in the spirit of birthing create an atmosphere that can give huge strength and confidence to the labouring woman.

There should be no talking during contractions, no bustling about or busyness, only a turning towards the woman in labour. She should be at the centre of everything that is happening, and her needs and wishes are paramount. If she wants to be alone, her helpers leave and wait near by. If she wants only one other person with her after all, that is her choice. There must be no conflict, no domineering attitudes, no competition to give her most help. Those present are simply watching and waiting on life.

supporting the midwife

It is vital that there is no friction between those present, and that there is at least one person in the group who quietly supports the midwife. This is especially the case in any country where home birth is perceived by most doctors as a dangerous gamble. The midwife may need somewhere to lie down and rest if labour is slow, may welcome food and drink and perhaps a bath. She also needs strong emotional support, and to know that her work is appreciated and that she is valued as a person.

An English midwife, Caroline Flint, has written: "To work as a midwife is stressful because, to work effectively and sensitively, the midwife gives so much of herself, and she becomes so involved with and such a part of the family with which she is involved. To enable her to be a fount of such strength, a source of so much comfort, she herself must have support and cherishing!"*

"I felt close to her. There was that wonderful 'with woman' feeling."

When one of my daughters was giving birth in our home, using a birth pool, the second stage was very gentle and was taking a long time. I was aware that both midwives were rather tired. I went to make a pot of tea to refresh us. The senior midwife came in and said, "Sheila, you are really confident that Tess can do this, aren't you?" We looked each other in the eyes. "Yes, I am. I have complete confidence in her." She smiled. "That's all right then," she replied, and went back to help the unfolding of this new life with increased confidence. It culminated in the triumphant birth in water of a 4.75 kg (10$\frac{1}{2}$lb) vigorous baby, whose mother had an intact perineum, and next to no bleeding. As Tess lifted him up in her arms, he looked up at her, turned to us, and then back to her, and smiled.

During those hours of labour there were two midwives, both dear friends of mine, Tess's husband Jon, myself, and my husband unobtrusively taking photographs. Tess clung to Jon physically, but with each late-first-stage contraction she sought the eyes of one midwife, while the other cradled her head in a way that made her feel utterly safe. At times one of us passed her a small sponge on which to suck, brushed her hair back from her face, or gave her iced water to sip. Sometimes I held her head and the midwife and Jon held her legs. Then Jon and I held her legs and the midwife her head. And when she was out of the water she often squatted or knelt, with the midwife and her husband on either side with their arms around her and the other midwife face to face with her, giving her understanding and love.

> "My three-year-old son saw his brother being born. When he saw the baby coming, he sang, 'Happy birthday to you'."

Afterwards the senior midwife told me that when she worked on the delivery suite in the hospital in the days following she felt very alone, even though midwives there are supposed to work as members of teams. Even in a large institution where people are milling about, and perhaps especially in a large institution, a midwife can feel unsupported. The support that other women can give a midwife in an out-of-hospital birth is precious.

children

Many women who already have children choose an out-of-hospital birth so that the older siblings can share in the birth experience, meet the new baby in an atmosphere that is warmer and more welcoming than that of a hospital, and do not have to be separated from their mother. Yet there is more to it even than that. All of us who approach childbirth with no idea of what happens except what can be gained from books and films, are deprived. Girls growing up without any awareness of what it feels like to give birth, other than the fear of pain and injury, are especially deprived. In medicalizing childbirth and removing it

> "There she was, wriggling and screaming! Chris lifted her into my arms. I realized my other three kids had missed her birth. Then there they were, in the room. Each of their faces, at that moment, is fixed in my mind for ever."

from the home, our culture has made birth, like dying, a fearful ordeal that can be dealt with only by experts, that is no longer part of our shared lives, and is out of women's control. In bringing birth back into a setting that is controlled by women, making it a family occasion, and involving the other children in the family, we reclaim it, and prepare children to reclaim it for themselves.

Women are often adamant that they would not want their older children present because it would be distracting and they would get in the way. They would have to be mothering when they wanted to concentrate on themselves. This is one effect of the isolation of women from each other. There is often no one else who understands what a small child wants or who can comfort him.

If your child is around when you are pushing the baby out, he is able to see what is happening, share in the excitement of birth, and touch and hold the new baby immediately afterwards. It will be an unforgettable experience.

"I agreed to look after Stephen (aged three) and take him out if he became bored. We went off and made gingerbread men in the kitchen, and then David called us back in because the baby was about to be born. She was pushing and we could soon see the crown of the baby's head. I explained what we were seeing and what was happening. With the next push the baby's head emerged. Stephen was enthralled! Soon after the baby was born, he sat in the armchair and cuddled her."

Remember that it is easy to overload a small child with information about birth and babies. This child wants to be the centre of your attention, and not feel rejected in favour of the new baby. So you will also want to talk about feelings: feeling alone, feeling loved, feeling excited, and feeling sad.

It is essential that your midwife knows your child too, so that she feels comfortable with the child's presence, and that the child knows her as a friend whose arrival is welcomed. They should have developed a relationship during the antenatal visits, when she explained what she was doing and why, in simple language, and got him to "help". Your older child will have already listened to the baby's heartbeats like galloping hooves, felt the baby kick, seen you practise the different positions and movements you may want to use in labour, and watched you relaxing and breathing.

A child at a home birth is witness to the care and love that is given to the mother. This is an important learning experience about human compassion, sensitivity, and tenderness. The child is witness also to the power in women, the energy in the mother,

"Olivia is seven and begged not to be left out of it. She was sitting beside me when the baby's head was born, and leant over and kissed it and said, 'Hello, baby!' I felt a wave of warmth and love for her and for everybody, and at the next push the baby slithered out. She was so excited! We all kissed and cuddled and cried with joy."

and the strength of women to help and support each other. And, if it turns out that way, the child is present as the miracle of life unfolds, hears the first cry, and sees warm, damp, crumpled flesh become a little person who can be held in her own arms and stroked.

Preparing your child

Q A What do I tell my child about birth?

Be completely open and honest about the birth and make it exciting. "The baby grows inside a muscle bag called 'the uterus'. When it is ready to be born my uterus squeezes tightly and gives the baby very big hugs. The opening of the bag gets bigger and bigger until the top of the baby's head can pass through, like when your head pushes through the neck of your sweater..."

Q A How else can I prepare my child?

It is a good idea to rehearse the noises you may make, so that the child is not surprised by them: grunting, moaning, panting, sighing and groaning. This can be great fun! Plan ahead and let the child share your plans. An older child can make his or her own birth plan, too: what to play with during labour, how to help you in simple ways, and what the party will be like after the baby is born.

Q A Should I ask someone to be there to look after my child?

Having a child around when you are in labour works only if someone whom he loves has special responsibility for the child. Otherwise your birth partner will be constantly distracted from attending to your needs with changing a nappy, fetching a potty, finding the teddy bear, or kissing a hurt better.

Q A Should my child watch the birth?

You know your child best. It depends a lot on your feelings at the time, too. Don't sit a two-year-old in front of you in labour and expect him to watch quietly if what he really wants is to stampede around the garden. He should be free to go in and out and cuddle up beside you when he wants the comfort of your presence or is sleepy.

Q A Could the experience be overwhelming?

Children usually take birth in their stride if they are well prepared and feel secure.

meeting challenges

All that is needed for most labours to go well is a healthy, pregnant woman who has loving support in labour, self-confidence, and attendants with infinite patience. Sadly most of us don't have these things, and then even a straightforward labour can become difficult, with rescue manoeuvres taking the place of the nurturing that is the basis of good midwifery care. Women who have their babies in hospital are more likely to have difficult labours because they are in hospital. The physiology of birth has been disturbed. They are also at risk of suffering the effects of iatrogenic medical care – that is, being subjected to interventions that themselves introduce pathology. This is not to say that problems never develop in planned out-of-hospital births, only that they can usually be solved by simple, non-invasive measures.

In this chapter I look what can be done when difficulties are encountered, so that you and your midwife can discuss together what action to take.

what if I'm overdue?

Most babies are not born on the date they are expected. Generally speaking, it is safer for them to be born after the expected date than preterm. Although with prolonged pregnancy every hour may seem like a week, and each week a month, a baby will usually be born within ten days of the expected date. If you go past ten days, it may be because you had a long menstrual cycle, ovulated later than you thought, and so conceived later, or because the date based on ultrasound that you were given was incorrect. Gestational age based on the known first day of the last menstruation is sometimes more accurate than ultrasound.*

"There is an unexplained stillbirth rate of one in 1,000 babies at 40 weeks. This starts to go up at 41 weeks, when it is 1.2 per 1,000 births. At 42 weeks it is 1.3 per 1,000 births. So there seems to be no advantage in inducing labour before 40 weeks unless the baby is obviously not doing well in the uterus."*

"Kathryn was originally due on 12 September, but she was born on 20 October. I was allowed to go for so long overdue as it was decided that I had not conceived until four weeks after my last period. I had only one period after coming off the Pill, and the cycle had not returned to normal."

Going for bumpy car rides or drinking gin does not start labour. Uncomfortable journeys just leave you tired and aching. Alcohol inhibits labour. Alcohol used to be given to stop preterm labour because it prevents secretion by the pituitary gland of oxytocin, the natural substance that initiates labour. It may cause respiratory depression in the newborn.*

Sexual arousal

You may find that contractions start after sexual stimulation, which leads to the release of oxytocin in the bloodstream. This may have an effect similar to that of synthetic oxytocin administered through an intravenous drip in order to start labour artificially. Even what is for many women the very gentle arousal produced by nipple stimulation, carried out by you or someone else, may produce contractions if continued for 20 minutes or so at a time.* Stroke the nipples with your fingers, rolling, sucking or licking them, or rest a warm face cloth on your breasts, lifting it off when it cools, dipping it in hot water, and pressing it against the nipples again.

Contractions may at first be very short, and gradually become longer, although in some women long, strong contractions are stimulated immediately. If they last for one minute or longer, reduce or stop the stimulation, since you may be particularly sensitive to it.

As you stimulate one nipple, you will notice that both nipples react, and may be aware of sensations in the other breast too. The same happens when you breastfeed. When the baby sucks at one breast, the milk ejection reflex occurs in both.

There is an extraordinary link between the nipples and the uterus, as you discover when you breastfeed. In the days after birth, when the baby latches on, you experience the warm, buzzing, milk ejection reflex as blood rushes into your breasts and, either at the same time, or soon after as the baby sucks, strong contractions of the uterus. These can be quite painful in the early days, but they are useful because they speed up your uterus's return to its pre-pregnancy size and shape.

Sexual intercourse may also stimulate contractions. This is because of the combined effect of oxytocin release and semen in the vagina. Semen is rich in prostaglandins. In fact, it is the richest source in the human body. Synthetic prostaglandins are used for induction in the form of a gel or pessary inserted in the cervix. To be most effective, semen should form a pool around the cervix. So back to the missionary position! Lie still for half an hour after your partner has ejaculated, so that the semen collects round the cervix. During this time your partner can caress your breasts so that you have both forms of stimulation.

Some years ago the Japanese invented a whirring machine that could be inserted against the cervix to start contractions, because it was found that local stimulation of the tissues was effective for induction. In the absence of such a machine, and perhaps in preference to it, you might explore the effect of lying on your back with your ankles on your partner's shoulders so that his penis can be introduced deeply. This is not comfortable and should be done very, very gently. A clean finger could be used to tickle the cervix gently instead.

"My doctor was muttering about induction. So we went to bed early and decided to try your method of natural induction. Contractions started, like cramps, about ten minutes after we made love, and Neil kept them going by playing with my nipples while I dozed off . . . I came to about three o'clock in the morning when contractions were coming about every five minutes. Neil was half-asleep but had one hand on the top of my tummy to feel contractions, and kept twiddling my nipple with the other. He felt very pleased with himself."

You can experience sexual arousal without a partner, of course. Masturbation will also produce contractions and, because it is possible to have an orgasm very quickly and to experience multiple orgasm, with self-stimulation, it may be a more effective method than intercourse in starting off labour.

Although breast or clitoral stimulation does not always get labour going, it may well ripen your cervix, making it soft, flexible, and thinned out, so that it dilates more easily when labour really does start properly.

Observing fetal movements

If you go past your due date, it may be reassuring to make a note of fetal movements. A baby who is moving vigorously is fine.

Although a baby makes fewer whole-body movements in the last few weeks of pregnancy, because it is a tight fit in the uterus, a healthy baby continues to kick, often when you are resting or lying in the bath. You can select a time of day when your baby is always at its most active and monitor what is happening during that time.

If you find that your baby has quietened down, the most likely possibility is that labour is about to start. There may be other signs:
♦ A rush of energy as you feel the "nesting" instinct and want to clean out cupboards or finish a work project.
♦ The need to empty your bladder frequently.
♦ Slight looseness of the bowels – like a minor digestive upset.
♦ Low backache.
♦ A feeling that your baby's head is hanging between your legs like a coconut.
♦ More frequent Braxton Hicks (practice) contractions of your uterus.

When movements are much reduced and labour does not start, there is a chance that a baby is no longer being nourished well by the placenta. You will want to check on this, so ring your midwife, say what has happened, and ask for fetal heart monitoring.

You can enjoy these last unanticipated days of pregnancy with special activities for which otherwise you will never have time – that restaurant you meant to try, the concert you thought you wouldn't be able to go to because the baby would just be born, a day with a friend, a picnic, a trip to an art gallery or museum, or a play or film that you can fit in now. Don't just sit and wait for the first twinges and brood over what seems by now to be an elephant pregnancy. Soon there will be a baby in your arms.

what if I think labour has started, but it hasn't?

Many women have painful contractions that might be the start of labour in the last few weeks before they actually go into labour. This is "prodromal" labour, and means that changes are taking place in preparation for labour before dilatation starts. It is a sign that contractions are beginning to soften and thin out the cervix and push down the baby's presenting part – the part of the baby nearest your cervix, usually the head. Although tiring, this may reduce the length of time you are in labour.

You may be told that you are in "false" labour. This does not mean that you are telling lies, or that your body is not working properly. What you are feeling is real. Contractions occur especially at night that may keep you awake, and may be quite regular for several hours. The problem with prodromal labour is that a woman is likely to be in a permanently alert state, waiting for further action. This is very tiring and results in a lowering of morale even before she feels regular contractions that dilate the cervix.

If this happens to you, it is important to get sleep, perhaps with a special bed-time ritual – soaking in a bath with lavender oil, and then having a hot milk drink , or a glass of wine, and listening to soothing music as you settle down.

what if my waters break before labour starts?

Ten per cent of women have premature rupture of the membranes at term (when the baby is due), and eight out of ten of these start labour spontaneously within 12 hours*, although sometimes a woman has to wait as long as 24 hours before it begins. Premature rupture is more likely when there have been vaginal examinations in the weeks preceding*, so this is a good reason for declining such examinations in the last weeks of pregnancy.

When your waters break, there may be a gush of fluid or a slow trickle. If there is only a dribble, it is probably the hind waters, the part of the bubble behind the baby's head, that are leaking, and they often reseal themselves. You can ignore it. If there is a gush of fluid, note whether it is clear, or stained brown or green. If it is clear, and your baby is engaged in your pelvis, you do not need to take special action. If it is stained, the baby has emptied its bowels of meconium, a sign that it could be under stress. Call your midwife so that the baby's position can be checked. Often meconium is not fresh, which is a sign that the baby was stressed some time ago. If your baby is breech, meconium is squeezed out mechanically as the bottom is pressed down. This is not an indication that the baby is stressed.

When you go into labour, the time spent getting to know and trust your midwife during the pregnancy prove to be invaluable.

Premature rupture of the membranes is sometimes taken as a sign that a woman is going to have a more difficult labour. But this is not so. There is no such thing as a "dry" labour, because fresh amniotic fluid is created that keeps the baby, its cord, and the surrounding tissues moist.

An important thing to know when membranes rupture is the position in which your baby is lying. So it is helpful to be aware of this at the end of pregnancy. If the baby is head down and the head is low in the pelvis, there is no possibility of the type of emergency occurring when a loop of cord slips down beneath the head (see page 140). There is a remote chance of this happening if the head is still high, however, or if the baby is lying in a less usual position – breech or transverse (across the uterus). Once your membranes have ruptured, do not put anything inside your vagina or you may introduce infection. There should be no vaginal examinations out of curiosity, either. The more vaginal examinations that take place, the greater the risk of infection.

If you wait anxiously for the first contraction, you will be tired out by the time your energy is really needed. So put on a sanitary pad – change it regularly – and go to bed and sleep, do some gentle work around the house or garden, play cards, or a good board game, listen to music, or watch television.

To check that there is no infection, take your temperature every three to four hours. If there is infection, you become slightly feverish, and you should let your caregiver know this. When you empty your bowels, be careful to wipe from front to back, away from your vagina, so that you do not introduce bacteria from your rectum. Don't starve yourself during this wait. You may not want to eat once labour starts, so avoid a long fast now. Have plenty of fluids – fruit juice, tea, or whatever you fancy – to help replace your amniotic fluid, and keep your energy up with snacks of high carbohydrate food, such as pasta, baked potato and pancakes with syrup. Some midwives suggest taking supplementary vitamin C to build resistance to infection, 250 mg every few hours*.

what if the cord prolapses?

A prolapsed cord is an obstetric emergency. It occurs rarely – in 0.3 per cent of pregnancies. It happens occasionally in late pregnancy, when membranes rupture prematurely, whether or not a woman intends to have her baby in hospital. Prolapse is dangerous because the baby's oxygen supply depends on blood flowing freely through the cord. When it prolapses, the cord gets nipped between the mother's pelvis and the baby's presenting part (head or bottom). A Caesarean section is often the only way to deliver the baby safely.

Your midwife will diagnose that the baby's cord is trapped if it can be felt pulsating in your vagina, but sometimes it is too high to feel, and the clue is a marked deceleration in the fetal heart immediately following membrane rupture when the presenting part was high. Go to hospital immediately.

Emergency treatment is to get into a knee-chest position with your bottom high in the air. Your midwife, or your birth partner if no professional caregiver is present, inserts two clean fingers in your cervix to press the baby's presenting part up and away from the cord. If you go to hospital in a car or ambulance, keep in this position with a blanket thrown over you, your pelvis raised high on a beanbag or pile of pillows, and your helper's fingers maintaining pressure inside your cervix to lift the presenting part away from it. An alternative is for her to introduce 400–700ml of saline into your bladder to cushion the cord. This slows down uterine activity for a while, too.

A prolapsed cord is very unlikely to occur during a home birth or in any birth place where invasive procedures are not practised. It is usually a consequence of intervention – rupturing the membranes artificially when the presenting part is high.

how can I handle a long, slow labour?

It is difficult to time the onset of labour precisely and, although some women are suddenly aware that this is IT, far more experience a gentle lead-in to labour. You may decide you are in labour with contractions that are spaced about ten minutes from the start of one to the start of the next, or may adopt a "wait and see" attitude. Anxiety makes a woman more sensitive to the pre-labour phase and alerts her to action before she can do anything to help herself. It is better to relax and let things happen. Your body will tell you that you are in labour when it really needs your concentrated attention.

"Ross and I decided to take the dog for a vigorous walk in the park to see if we could hurry things along. It was a real pleasure, interrupted by strong contractions that began coming every ten minutes again. I sat down, or leaned against him or a tree, and he supported me through the breathing. I felt strong and confident."

The shortest labours are not necessarily the best. A rapid labour can be shocking for the mother and prove stressful for the baby. In statistical terms the best outcomes follow a labour of between 12 and 24 hours for women having their first babies, and a labour lasting between 3 and 24 hours for women having subsequent babies.*

Slow dilatation is completely normal for some women. The arbitrary decision made by obstetricians who practise "active management" that labour must not last longer than 12 hours, or that dilatation must proceed by 1 cm per hour, puts the woman under stress and makes her attendants anxious too, so that they sometimes act unwisely in an attempt to hurry labour along. They may rupture the membranes in order to hasten a slow

Woman having a hospital birth:

"If someone doesn't cover that clock, I'm going to break it!"

labour. But if this is done before 4 cm dilatation of the cervix, it can actually slow down labour that is already progressing at a slow rate. If you are already around 9cm dilated, however – the point at which membranes usually rupture naturally – amniotomy may speed up the late first stage.*

In hospital a long, slow labour is often termed "failure to progress" only because caregivers find the waiting intolerable. There is an art in adapting to a long labour and not being hassled or discouraged.

♦ Intersperse activity and rest, and change your activities frequently. Avoid boredom. Bake a cake for the celebration afterwards, soak in a bath, go for a walk, sew or knit – anything rather than lying in bed wondering if there is something wrong because labour is not going faster.

♦ Eat easily digested, smooth foods, such as potato puree, soup, mashed banana, ice-cream, sorbet, honey sandwiches, or yogurt, and drink plenty of fluids. In most cultures special foods are used to keep up a woman's strength. In Pakistan it may be a paste of dates and sesame seeds; in China chicken ginger soup; in Colombia fig juice; and in the Caribbean spice tea which, like the raspberry leaf tea that is popular in Europe, has a mild oxytocic action.

♦ Move around and keep changing position to stimulate uterine activity, and to encourage the baby to descend and rotate with the crown of the head against your cervix. Rock your pelvis, go up and down stairs, and lunge against the wall.

♦ Soak in a bath or have a shower to refresh you and help you to relax your mind and body.

♦ Empty your bladder every hour and a half to two hours. (Your partner can keep a note of it and remind you.)

♦ A woman in slow labour welcomes quiet, calm reassurance: "You are doing well. The baby is fine. It doesn't matter that labour is slow." You should not feel under any pressure of time. It is often good to be left alone with your birth partner.

♦ Explore what happens when you do nipple stimulation or gentle clitoral massage. You can do it yourself or ask your partner to do it. Or you could both get into bed, send everyone away, turn off the light, and have a cuddle for an hour.

A midwife discussing a client's labour:

"We spent much of the first stage in the garden, putting in bedding plants together. Then we came in and made some biscuits and cleared up the kitchen. By that time, I could tell from her breathing that she was nearly fully dilated."

"Contractions stopped completely. I was so disappointed. I felt ready to cry. So I did cry, long and hard. John and I barbecued the biggest steak we could find and ate lots of salad and vegetables and potatoes to keep it company. I put an apple-sauce cake in the oven and got ready for bed. Then I felt a strong contraction and, after that, another one . . ."

"I lay down for a couple of hours, and my contractions spaced out more. Then I got up again and found that, with walking, the intensity increased and they came every three or four minutes, lasting 45 to 60 seconds."

what if I have a start-stop labour?

Some labours are slow in a different way. They start and then seem to stop. The uterus contracts weakly or ceases to contract for an interval, then starts again, but may have another phase of inactivity. There may be plateaux like this when nothing much seems to be happening.

A start-stop labour occurs most commonly when a woman is admitted to hospital and her previous regular, strong contractions become spasmodic and weak. The cause is anxiety. The uterus is very responsive to anxiety and this is as true for other mammals as for women. Interference can make any animal's labour more difficult. For example, when mice are disturbed during labour, their labours are prolonged and they are more likely to deliver dead pups.*

> "Everything got very quiet, with gentle contractions like ripples. I felt drowsy and dreamy. Nothing seemed to be happening. I wondered if I'd know when to push. But there was no doubt about it. After about half an hour I suddenly felt this great wave of longing and incredible rush of energy and I shouted, 'Got to push!'."

If you have a start-stop labour, try to find why you are anxious. Bring it out into the open, and ask your birth partner and midwife to help you deal with it. Before you can melt into your labour, you are going to have to discard all these fears.

Keep active, unless you are very tired, in which case rest in a darkened room, perhaps with soft music to screen you from any disturbing sounds. Your midwife can rest near you, and many midwives bring some sewing or other work to do ready for just such eventualities.

There is a physical cause for some start-stop labours. The baby's head is in an awkward position and becomes stuck. Your midwife will monitor the fetal heart regularly and assess the situation. When a baby is awkwardly positioned, moving about and rocking and rolling your pelvis may coax it into a better position so that labour can progress. And even when the head is a tight fit, and the baby's descent through the pelvis is delayed, the spontaneous movements a woman makes can assist the uterus to ease the baby's head through the cervix and down the birth canal.

The diagnosis of cephalo-pelvic disproportion (CPD) is made far too often, when what is really meant is, "We couldn't be bothered to wait," or "We were afraid," or "The mother's morale dropped," or "She got very tired." If after discussion and exploring alternative ways of stimulating labour you decide that further action is called for, you will need to transfer to hospital. An oxytocin intravenous drip (syntocinon) cannot be set up at home because it is a powerful and potentially dangerous drug. For some labours it is the most effective solution to reduced uterine activity. This situation is not an emergency, however, and you will have sufficient time to discuss the options fully and come to a decision with your midwife.

if there is a lull at the end of the first stage, how should we handle it?

When the baby's head is high and still above the level of the ischial spines – the bony protruberances in the pelvic cavity – there is often a pause at the very end of the first stage of labour. The uterus rests, and everyone else can rest too. In hospital, during this pause, the decision is often made to set up a syntocinon drip in order to stimulate the uterus into action.

It is wiser to wait for descent and rotation of the head to occur, and give your body a chance to prepare for the active second stage. You can use what I call the "rest and be thankful" phase to good advantage – perhaps have a shower – and come out of it refreshed and with renewed energy.

The pushing reflex

Squatting is a good position for initiating contractions and encouraging rotation of the baby's head so that it can press against your pelvic floor muscles. When the head touches nerves in these muscles, the pushing reflex is stimulated, and oxytocin spurts into your bloodstream, causing strong contractions. If you start pushing simply because you are fully dilated and have been told to do so, but do not feel the spontaneous reflex, you may become exhausted with straining, and are likely to push the baby's head down unrotated, with resulting deep transverse arrest, when the baby cannot turn its head to the easiest position for delivery. In most labours this is avoidable if a woman is not urged to push too soon and if everyone waits patiently.

how can I deal with backache?

One of the most difficult things to handle in labour is low backache. It continues as a gnawing ache between contractions, as well as being a sharp sacro-lumbar pain during them, and can wear down any woman's spirits. Backache occurs particularly when the baby's back is against the mother's spine (posterior position), and the hard back of the baby's extended head (that is, when the chin is lifted) is pressing against her sacrum and sacrolumbar ligaments. Any position in which the baby is tipped forwards on to the mother's abdominal wall and away from her spine may ease it: a forward-kneeling or all-fours position, for example, together with swinging, rocking, and circling of the pelvis. Tipping the baby forwards also helps it to rotate from the posterior to the anterior position, since it is easier for the baby to tuck its head in and turn against the abdominal muscles, especially if they are relaxed, than against the bony spine.

"It was painful. My midwives told me that they knew it was hard for me but that the baby was fine. That made all the difference."

Firm massage or counter-pressure over the painful area is also helpful. Hot or cold compresses relieve pain too. Either a hot-water bottle or a small packet of frozen peas may work well. A strong jet of hot or cold water directed on to the spot as pain builds up often brings relief. Some women labouring in water find that massage while they are in a forward-leaning position in the pool provides amazing pain-relief.

Transcutaneous electronic nerve stimulation (TENS) helps some women, but proves irritating or ineffective for others. TENS is done with a hand-held instrument, about the size of a small camera, which sends electrical impulses to the brain to block pain messages. It is battery-operated, with four electrodes which are attached with adhesive tape at either side of the spine, two with their upper edges at the level of the lower ribs and two in the lower back. You control its operation yourself and can move about, lie down, or sit up. It seems to be less effective for abdominal than for back pain.

The instrument's low-frequency current produces a buzzing sensation, which stimulates the release of endogenous (natural) opiates and endorphins into the cerebro-spinal fluid, thus raising tolerance of pain and increasing the sense of wellbeing.* If you know before the onset of labour that your baby is posterior, it can be worth getting hold of TENS equipment. It is something you can do to help yourself, and is harmless to the baby.*

Any woman with severe backache needs her helpers' undivided attention, and encouragement to keep going. Because pain of this kind is very wearing, she may feel unable to move about. If this happens to you, flop forwards, spreadeagled over a beanbag, so that your partner can reach your back and massage or press against it. The position will help the baby's head to rotate. Or lie on your side with your underneath arm spread out behind you, your limbs well flexed, and your head bent forwards. You will spontaneously select the correct – because more comfortable – side on which to lie. Most posterior babies lie with the back on the mother's right: the right occipito posterior (ROP) position. This is five times more common than left occipito posterior (LOP). If your baby is ROP, lie on your left side with your top knee drawn up and pressing against your abdomen. This encourages the baby to tip forwards into a position where it is easier for it to turn to the anterior. If your baby is LOP, you will be more comfortable on your right side, and this helps the baby turn.

> "The three hours that transition lasted seemed endless. 'When will this be over?' I kept muttering. The pain no longer seemed localized low in my abdomen. It overtook my whole body. It was huge and overwhelming."

If this position, your birth partner can sit close against your lower back, with the side of his pelvis pressing hard against the area where you feel most pain. Experiment to find the right spot. Then you can have the whole weight of his body against you at the peak of pain. He can also massage your back by rocking his pelvis.

Once the baby rotates, backache may vanish almost miraculously, and you go straight into the pushing stage. When I was doing anthropological field work in Jamaica, I found that the shape of many women's pelvises was such that their babies were posterior for a long time in labour. They disliked the backache but welcomed it as a sign that the "gate" in their backs was creaking open to let the baby out. If you think of that pain as a gate opening, it may be easier to bear. Once it is open wide, you know that the baby is almost with you.

what if I feel I can't go on?

Most women feel that they can't go on and would like to postpone having the baby when they reach the end of the first stage of labour. These feelings are a sign of progress: for this is transition, the bridge between the first and second stage. You long for some rest from the storm of contractions and may get very irritable. In a long labour, or one with backache, you are likely to feel discouraged earlier than this. The words used, and the tone in which they are said, are of first importance. There is no formula that is right for every woman. But a good midwife has phrases that express her conviction that the woman can do it, in a way that is sympathetic and empowering.

I can almost hear my friend Caroline Flint murmuring encouraging words – similar to the ones I often find myself using when I am with a woman in labour:

Good . . . Excellent . . . You're doing so well . . . You're beautifully relaxed . . . Let it happen . . . Let it come . . . Let it open you up . . . Surrender to it . . . Feel yourself opening up . . . Good, good, good. Well done . . . That's wonderful . . . That's marvellous . . . Oh, how brilliant . . . That's lovely . . . Blossom . . . Flourish . . . Open up to it . . . Be soft . . . Be giving . . . Surrender to it . . . Give, give, give . . . Surrender . . . Open, open . . . Good . . . Good, good . . .*

However tired she is, the midwife should never use these words mechanically. They express her inner awareness that the woman needs to release all tension, find her body's rhythms, and open wide.

Elizabeth Davis, midwife in San Francisco, uses such phrases as: "Keep it loose," and "Be really open and let that force move through you, just let it be, let it down."*

Penny Simkin, a childbirth educator in Seattle, has what she calls the "take charge routine" for any time in labour when a woman hits an emotional low, weeps, wants to give up, is very tense, or is in a great deal of pain. The birth partner or midwife moves in close to the mother to help her regain her inner strength. She speaks in a calm, confident voice, as she says:

Breathe with me . . . BREATHE WITH ME . . . That's the way . . . just like that . . . Good . . . STAY WITH IT . . . just like that . . . LOOK AT ME . . . Stay with me . . . Good for you . . . It's going away

. . . Good . . . Good . . . Now just rest, that was so good.

Between contractions she may say:

With the next one let me help you more. I want you to look at me the moment it starts. We will breathe together so it won't get ahead of us. Okay? Good, you're doing so well. We're really moving now.*

If there comes a time in labour when you are discouraged, you need change. You can change what you are doing, or your environment.

♦ Change your position or the movements you are making.

♦ If you have background music, change the CD and select a completely different rhythm or mood.

♦ Have a change of scene. Move to another room or out-of-doors. Open the window or go to the bathroom.

♦ Try changing the rhythm of your breathing. If you were tending to breathe fast, now breathe more slowly and fully. If you were breathing deeply, let your breathing speed up and allow it to "dance" a little.

♦ Ask for a change in the kind of touch you are receiving, on a different place on your body, or a different kind of massage. Have your helpers switch over so that you are held or massaged by someone else.

♦ If other people to whom you feel close are available, ask one of them to come and be with you for a while. A fresh face often works wonders.

♦ If you have been in semi-darkness, now light a lot of candles or turn the lights up. If the room is bright, draw the curtains or dim the lights.

♦ Change the essential oils in your oil burner or choose a different massage oil, from lavender to rose, from frankincense to juniper or orange, for example.

♦ If you have had your eyes closed during contractions, open them now, and make eye contact with your birth partner or your midwife. If you have been in eye contact until now, try closing your eyes and sinking down into yourself near the source of the power released deep in your body.

♦ Perhaps you have been silent during your contractions until now. You could try opening yourself up and making low sounds that go right down into your pelvis. Or, if you have been making a great deal of noise, now is the time to listen to the sound of your own breathing during contractions, and let each breath sound like a wave on the shingle.

♦ Freshen up. Splash your face with cold water. Get someone to brush your hair back slowly from your face. Have a bath or shower. Suck cracked ice.

♦ Pep up your energy with a glucose drink or spoonfuls of honey eaten from the pot.

the drive to control your body

It is often claimed that dancers and horse-riders have hard labours because their pelvic floor muscles are thick. But a well-exercised muscle is also a flexible muscle. It can be contracted or released at will. The problem is more likely to be that a woman who dominates her body with stamina and courage can fight her labour longer. Muscular exertion will not help her in childbirth. She needs to surrender control of her muscles so her uterus can work for her.

Ina May Gaskin, midwife at the alternative-style community, The Farm, in Tennessee, describes attending a cyclist who had already been in labour for 24 hours and was becoming discouraged. She says:

I was pretty sure that her problem had been that, in not really "welcoming" each rush, she was actually fighting labor in a subtle but effective way.

Then I asked her what had been the longest she had ever ridden her bicycle in one day. She looked at her husband, and together they said, "120 miles", and smiled. I said, "Having a baby is a lot like that. It takes endurance. But you have to learn a different way of pedalling." That seemed to make sense to her. I explained that she needed to be aware of the sensations that came with each rush and try to help open up and relax when each one came. I suggested that smooching would often aid the process. I left them alone for approximately 45 minutes, after which they called me back to check her dilation. By this time she was nearly fully dilated and was about to begin spontaneous pushing. She loved pushing and delivered her baby quite easily without a tear.*

Labour is like swimming in a stormy sea. Go with the current.

what if the midwife is worried about the fetal heart-rate?

If the baby's heart-rate slows as a contraction reaches its peak, it should pick up again by about 15 seconds after the end of a contraction. If it does this, the baby is receiving sufficient oxygen.

The easiest way for your midwife to monitor this in an out-of-hospital labour is by using Doppler ultrasound, a sonic aid held against your abdomen over the baby's heart, to listen intermittently to the heart for 30 seconds following a contraction. The sonic aid can be used, whatever your position, even under water if it is in a polythene bag or a condom. It leaves you free to move and, because you also hear the sound, keeps you, as well as the midwife, informed.

If the fetal heart slows to below 100 beats per minute and does not recover in the interval between contractions, this baby may be finding it hard-going. The problem may be that the cord has been pressed between the baby and your pelvis, and this can be solved if you change position. If you have been sitting or lying down, try a standing or all-fours position. If you are already in the second stage and have been holding your breath to push, try breathing instead, keeping your throat open. This is difficult if you are already in a pattern of breath-holding. It may help to blow out when the urge to push comes. Sometimes the baby just needs you to breathe more regularly, to keep on taking in oxygen, to have an easier birth. Your midwife will be carrying oxygen in case the baby needs a whiff after birth, and may have an oxygen mask for you to use at this point.

If, despite all your efforts, transfer to hospital is suggested, it is not failure. You have managed well up to this stage, but now need the extra help that the hospital can provide.

Once in hospital, continuous electronic fetal monitoring may be carried out, with an electrode attached to the baby's scalp. Although this provides a continuous print-out, it is impossible to diagnose fetal distress accurately from it. One way of obtaining further information is to prick the baby's scalp and take a few drops of blood to be analysed. On the basis of the result you may be advised to have a forceps or vacuum extraction delivery or a Caesarean section. Or the doctors may think that it is "better to be safe than sorry" and decide, without further investigation, to deliver the baby immediately by one of these methods. This will be a shock but, after all your hard work, it may be what you want too, or you may want to discuss it further and wait a bit.

what's the best way to deal with hyperventilation?

Hyperventilation is the result of breathing fast and furiously. It often happens at the end of the first stage, when contractions are coming at two-minute intervals. The woman breathes too heavily, and allows no time for the slight pauses that come naturally between inspiration and expiration and between expiration and inspiration. She feels light-headed, giddy, and nauseous, has tingling fingers, is numb around the mouth, starts to sweat, and may feel terribly panicky. Physiologically she has an increased pulse rate, a rise in blood pH (which means that the blood becomes more acidic) and blood flow to her brain decreases. A healthy baby copes well with a mother's over-breathing in labour, but a baby who is not in such good condition could be harmed by this flushing out of carbon dioxide because, when this occurs, oxygen is more firmly bound to haemoglobin and cannot be easily extracted by the cells. As a result the baby gets less oxygen.*

People often hyperventilate when under stress. Labour, especially the late first stage, is stressful. It may help if, as each contraction reaches a peak, your midwife or birth partner says: "Half way there," or "It'll soon be over now," and uses touch to give you confidence and comfort.

You can avoid hyperventilating by keeping your shoulders and throat relaxed, by focusing on the idea of relaxing a little more with each breath out, and by letting your breathing flow rhythmically. Your helpers can breathe with you so that you do not feel so alone.

If you hyperventilate, your partner can rest both hands on your shoulders and ask you to relax them and breathe more gently, with a slow sigh out. If you find this hard to do, it may help to breathe into a paper bag so that you can inhale the carbon dioxide you have exhaled. As you do this, focus on the short pause after each breath in and each breath out.

what if I get very tired?

Labour is an intense, energy-consuming activity. It may be the most strenuous work you have ever done. A woman often feels as if she is on a treadmill of contractions. The suggestions listed on page 157 will be useful now.

In some hospitals there is still a rule that a woman in labour must not eat anything, because of the danger of aspirating the contents of her stomach if she were to have a general anaesthetic. This can happen largely because gastric emptying is delayed when a woman has narcotic drugs – pethidine, for example – to relieve pain. Her only chance of being fed is through glucose and fluids via an intravenous drip. A labouring woman is bound to be exhausted if she is starving, especially if she is vomiting too. She has to draw on her fat reserves for energy, with the result that she becomes dehydrated and ketones, produced by metabolization of fat, appear in her urine.*

"After five hours I was beginning to tire of riding the pains. Anne was encouraging me all the time, saying: 'Relax into it – you're doing very well – very good.' She put a sponge in my mouth and I sucked on it, and she wiped my face with a warm, damp flannel. She said to me: 'Don't worry about other people. Just breathe. Keep breathing. You are doing it. You've made it. Well done!' The midwife said I was only 5-6 cm dilated. Anne said, 'You know it goes much more quickly from now on.' "

A woman having her baby in an out-of-hospital setting is unlikely to have analgesics that delay gastric emptying and can drink when she wishes and eat according to her appetite. So ketosis occurs less often in birth at home. But if labour is very tiring, here are some simple remedies:

♦ Have a drink to adjust your body's electrolyte balance such as "Labor-Aid".* This drink has been devised by American home birth midwives specifically for women in labour.

You make it by mixing together 1 quart water, $\frac{1}{3}$ cup honey, $\frac{1}{3}$ cup lemon juice, $\frac{1}{2}$ teaspoon salt, $\frac{1}{4}$ teaspoon baking powder and 2 crushed calcium tablets.

♦ Eat something that will just slip down. You may fancy frozen yoghurt or fromage frais, some smooth porridge with honey or syrup, or a few spoonfuls of mashed mango. These will give you instant energy.

♦ Do not fight the pain. Go right into it instead. Resisting it means that you are not allowing your body to open up. A surprising release can come when we accept pain and go with it.

♦ Whatever happens during contractions, rest completely in each interval between. Drop forwards on to pillows. It is often possible to sleep for half a minute before the next contraction starts. Ask your birth partner to rest a hand on your abdomen and tell you softly when the next one is starting, so that you can tune in to it and not be taken by surprise.

♦ Remember that you are having a baby. It is easy to forget this in the thick of labour. One midwife friend of mine often borrows a baby to bring to the woman in labour when she is at this stage, to remind her of what it is all about. A birth partner or a midwife says: "Come on, baby! Come on down. Come on, baby – just a little more." This may give you fresh heart.

what should I do if I want to push before I'm fully dilated?

You may have the desire to push before your cervix is fully open. Pushing hard against an incompletely dilated cervix can make it puffy and swollen so that it closes a little. This must make labour more difficult for the baby. If you want to push and are not yet 10 cm dilated, you may find the following suggestions helpful:

♦ Continue breathing. Do not hold your breath. When the longing to push comes, give two quick breaths out followed by one slow breath out, so that there is a steady rhythm of pant, pant, blow, breathe in. It sometimes helps if your birth partner holds up a finger in front of your mouth, so that you can direct each blow on to it. As soon as the urge leaves you, breathe fully and easily again.

♦ If you are in an upright position, change it and lie down on your side or be on all fours. This slightly reduces the pressure of the head against your rectum and anus, so you don't feel so desperate to push.

♦ If you have to push, do so with an open mouth and breathing out. Let your uterus do the work while you open up.

what if I don't get an urge to push?

A woman can have a baby without deliberately pushing it out. Her uterus sees to that. The energy that she gives to expulsion is only a small part – 30–40 per cent – of the power that is exerted by her uterus to press the baby down through the cervix, the folds of her vagina, and the spreading tissues of her perineum.

Until there is an irresistible urge to push, avoid pushing by continuing to breathe. There is no need to hold your breath at all. In this way, tissues have a chance to fan out smoothly before the ball of the baby's head eases through, with no damage to ligaments, muscles, or skin.

It feels marvellous to push when you want to, and you will know exactly how to do it. When you push instinctively the second stage is a triumphant experience.

Many women and birth attendants hope to hurry the birth along by pushing before the mother's body is quite ready. This can only do harm, and it is very tiring. Commanded pushing is distressing and exhausting, and often counter-productive because it makes the woman lose touch with what her body is telling her. It tends to turn the second stage into a prize fight, in which she is struggling to push the baby out, blood vessels bursting in her face and eyes, and blood pressure mounting, surrounded by supporters cheering her on, regardless of her spontaneous physiological rhythms. Imagine having people encouraging you while you were making love and you will see why it is not helpful. Imposing rules on a natural physiological activity that should be spontaneous is never a good idea.

"Then came the crowning. As quickly as this rush of contractions came, it stopped. I felt hot and high. I was excited. After climbing a very high mountain, I could now sit and enjoy the exhilarating view. I love this part of labour – the calm, high, ready feeling. My next contraction began, and I greeted it with satisfaction. Surprised by its intensity, I let my body do it."

Once the baby's head touches nerves in your perineum, the Ferguson reflex is stimulated, endogenous oxytocin is released, and you want to push.*

For some women this desire to push does not happen until the baby is just about to be born. The mother pushes once or twice and the baby slips out easily.

Sometimes the desire to push is there, but it is not strong. That's fine too. Go with your body. "Listen" to your uterus. When the second stage has started passionately, some gentler contractions may follow in which the pushing urge is faint or non-existent. For a woman who is free to follow her uterus, the pushing rhythm may vary with different contractions. Some pushes are short and others long. Sometimes there is only one push with a contraction, at other times four or five. Even if you feel unsure about what to do, your body knows how to give birth.

what if the second stage is taking a long time?

If you feel you have the strength to carry on, and the baby is doing well, setting a time limit on the second stage is totally unnecessary. Try and take one contraction at a time and relax completely between the contractions. The second stage of labour may last for three minutes or three hours and still be just the right amount of time required for that particular mother and baby.

what if the baby passes meconium?

The bowels of a mature fetus contain meconium. Meconium is a sign of maturity. Thick meconium passed at the beginning of labour means that the baby has been stressed, before labour started. If the baby inhales it, there is a chance of respiratory-tract infection.

Meconium is brown and sticky when fresh, green when stale. The passage of stale meconium is a sign that the baby may have been stressed in the past. If the baby is about to be born and fresh meconium is passed, your midwife or doctor will have a mucus extractor ready to suck out meconium gently – even before the baby's body is born, and before the chest has expanded to take the first breath.

It will be easier to do this if you stand with your knees bent or are on all fours, with your midwife or doctor behind you. Breathe the baby out gently, rather than pushing, and there will be time for your caregiver to suction out every bit of meconium.*

If you are nowhere near giving birth when the baby passes meconium, your birth attendants will probably suggest that you transfer to hospital so that a paediatrician can be ready to resuscitate a "flat" baby and make sure that the airways are clear by suctioning out any contents, using an endotracheal tube if necessary. "Flat" does not refer to a baby's shape when it is born, but to the level of vitality at birth. A "flat" baby appears limp and floppy, and breathing is depressed.

You may feel frightened about the need for transfer. Most babies who have passed meconium during labour are perfectly all right, but having a paediatric check-up and making sure that the baby's respiratory tract is clear means that you take no chances.

how can I cope if the baby is coming very fast?

When the second stage is rapid – a precipitate second stage – and it looks as if the baby will pop out like a champagne cork, there are several things you can do to slow the pace and make the birth gentler:

♦ Adopt an all-fours position, or lie on your side, so that your midwife can "guard" your perineum with a hand. Do not squat or stand.

♦ *Breathe* the baby out. Guide your baby down with your breathing. Avoid pushing. If you have to push, breathe again as soon as possible.

♦ Release your pelvic floor muscles and relax your perineum, by opening your mouth, dropping your jaw, and opening your glottis. Imagine a ripe fruit with all its seeds spilling out, or even a tube of toothpaste that you have accidentally stood on, with the toothpaste oozing out, or perhaps a waterfall with a great rush of water pouring through the rocks – whatever image best helps you relax.

♦ If you want to make noises you can moo, bellow, groan, or give deep sighs. The sounds should be resonant and go right down into your pelvis. Do not scream or yelp. That will make you tighten up.

♦ Release tension and open up, letting your pelvic floor descend like a lift down to the basement, rather than holding your breath and pushing deliberately. Then your baby can glide out, without being forcibly ejected.

> **A midwife*:**
>
> "Sometimes, while helping a mother through crowning, I feel like I'm outside a semitrailer truck, directing the driver: 'All right, bring it on a little now – hold it for a few seconds now. Okay, bring it on some more. While she holds back that tremendous force, the whole quality of her skin will change – she will relax and become more pliant and stretchy."

> "It all happened so fast – it was all over in less than an hour. I reached hospital at 3.15 p.m. and the midwife said I was 2 cm dilated. While she was examining me, I went to 5, and the baby was born at 3.50 p.m. I felt steam-rollered. I was shaking so much afterwards. I had to get up at 3 a.m. and write down what had happened to get it out of my system before I could settle to sleep."

If you don't want to miss the actual birth, remember to open your eyes and reach out your arms as soon as you feel the baby finally slither from your body.

what happens if the baby is a surprise breech?

Occasionally labour is going well and the birth attendants see something emerging that looks like a very bald head, and realize, perhaps after meconium is squeezed out, that it must be the baby's bottom. It is an undiagnosed breech.

Breech labour is like any other labour up to the point when the baby's body slips out. What may then happen is that the head gets stuck, which is why in hospitals when a breech is delivered vaginally – and many are delivered by Caesarean section – a large episiotomy is done and forceps are applied to the after-coming head. Actually most damage results from anxiety and rough handling by the person who is delivering. I have seen a doctor become anxious and pull on the baby's legs, so that the arms extended and the baby was completely stuck. A breech baby should always be delivered gently to avoid injury to the spinal cord, arms and neck.

Left to itself, the baby's body uncurls, the uterus keeps the head flexed, and one or both legs drop out, followed by the body and then the head. In a series of 89 breech births delivered by midwives in New Jersey, USA, there was no single case of extended arms, and all the babies were fine.*

It is unwise to plan a breech delivery at home, because your baby may need help to breathe, and a paediatrician should be available. But if you have a surprise breech, adopt a supported, upright position, legs wide apart and knees bent, in order to give the baby's head most space, and to enable gravity to help it slip through. Michel Odent says that he would "never risk a breech delivery with the mother in a dorsal or semi-seated position".*

The worst position for a breech delivery is lying on your back with legs raised in lithotomy stirrups, as most hospitals recommend. In that position your sacrum and coccyx are pressed up and the dimensions of your pelvic cavity and outlet are reduced. If you squat, however, you gain an extra centimetre across your pelvic cavity and two centimetres from front to back.*

Once you have adopted a half-standing, half-squatting position, leaning on your birth partner in front of you, your midwife should be positioned behind you, and simply wait and watch until the baby's body is completely born. The only intervention that may be necessary is to press gently behind the baby's knees if the feet are up over the shoulders. This will stimulate the baby to bend the knees so that they come down. When the legs are extended, they splint the spine, so that it is more difficult for the baby to take the curve of the birth canal.

As you bend your knees and go into a deep squat, holding on to your birth partner, the baby's body will slip out. The cord may slide down too, and if it is wrapped tightly around the baby, your midwife will carefully unloop it, but only very gently, or it may go into spasm. You may feel a confusing, intermittent pushing urge. Avoid pushing if you can until the head is ready to emerge. Let the baby be born by uterine activity alone. This will enable everything to open up and your tissues to spread wide. As soon as the whole body is born, drop forwards, legs still wide apart and knees bent, leaning over some furniture or your birth partner so that your back is almost horizontal. This tilts your pelvis so that the baby's nose and mouth are visible, and whoever is catching the baby can aspirate the nose and mouth with a mucus extractor before the head is fully born. A breech baby often begins to breathe once its chest is born, and may inhale mucus from your birth canal. The mucus can block the nasal passages, and although most babies are clever at sneezing out anything that is irritating, in this case aspiration is a wise precaution.

The decision has to be made as to whether or not to perform an episiotomy. Sometimes it is necessary in order to give the head more space to be born.

Then you will feel the crowning, with the sensation of heat and prickling that normally precede the birth, as the widest part of the baby's head passes over your perineum.

Your midwife may wrap a warm towel around the baby's body and support the head as it slides out. A breech baby may need a few whiffs of oxygen and some massage to recover from the shock of the birth.

should I have an episiotomy?

Although it is sometimes claimed that routine episiotomy rescues babies from cerebral trauma, there is no evidence for this. Randomised trials of births in which episiotomy was performed routinely or was used only when it was considered absolutely necessary reveal that no more babies have low Apgar scores or have to be sent to the special care nursery in the restricted episiotomy group.

A severe tear is more likely to occur when an episiotomy is performed than when a woman tears naturally. As an episiotomy heals it may be difficult to walk and sit. Many women say that it feels like sitting on jagged glass. Sometimes the episiotomy wound becomes infected, and women are more likely to have urinary incontinence and find any attempt at intercourse painful after episiotomy than after a natural tear.*

Unless the baby needs to be delivered quickly, it seems sensible to decline the offer of an episiotomy.

what can we do if there is shoulder dystocia?

When a baby is vertex (head down), sometimes a big head is born, and then there is a delay in the delivery of the shoulders. Very rarely the shoulders really are stuck. This is known as shoulder dystocia. The midwife can see that the baby's head is large, the cheeks are fat, and the face looks squashed. There is no sign of the neck, because it is wedged inside by the broad shoulders.

Shoulder dystocia may occur because the woman has had oxytocin stimulation of the uterus which has produced artificially strong contractions that have forced the pace, propelling a big baby along the birth canal before all the tissues have fanned out. The head shoots out, and the shoulders are impacted. Women giving birth out of hospital never have labour stimulated with oxytocin, so labour tends to be slower and gentler.

Deliberate forceful pushing with prolonged breath-holding may also eject a baby's head before the tissues have fanned out sufficiently, and because of this the shoulders are a tight fit. It seems better to allow labour to proceed at its own pace.

The head is the largest part of the baby and like a ball that can turn on the shoulders. When the baby is nestled down, back rounded, limbs flexed, and chin tucked in, the body is like a ball too. The head can rotate and move more or less independently of the body because of the neck, and the shoulders can rotate more or less independently of the head. If big shoulders are square on, the shoulders need to rotate so that first one can slip out, then the other.

Hospital doctors employ a range of techniques to deal with shoulder dystocia. These include pressure over the woman's pubis, a large episiotomy, fundal pressure applied over the baby's bottom, the

Wood "screw" manoeuvre that entails pushing the fingers inside and then pulling the baby out with a screwing motion, and the "Zavanelli manoeuvre", which involves pushing the head back in again and then delivering the baby by Caesarean section.*

If your baby's head is born and then nothing happens, move! Movement often releases the shoulders. Your birth partner can help you change position. Your midwife may ask you to get on hands and knees. The antero-posterior diameter (from front to back) of your pelvis increases by as much as one or two centimetres in this position. When the next contraction comes, push hard as your helper applies gentle downwards traction to the head. The baby sometimes falls out.*

Or stand with your knees as wide apart as possible. Caroline Flint believes that it probably does not matter exactly how a woman moves her pelvis, "from lying down to hands and knees; from kneeling to standing up; from standing up to being on all fours – but it is important for the movement to include a tilting of the pelvis".* This pelvic tilt occurs automatically when you bend one knee to get up into a standing position, stride forwards, or get down on the floor.

If your baby still does not budge, your helper will reach in with two fingers and find the baby's posterior armpit, the one nearest, and either pull the shoulder forwards or pull down the arm. Ina May Gaskin says that a colleague safely delivered a 6.25 kg (14 lb) baby in this way. She considers that episiotomy is usually unnecessary.

what happens if the midwife suddenly finds it's twins?

The mother of twins is more likely to develop high blood pressure and pre-eclampsia, and twins are at greater risk than singleton babies, especially the second baby. The babies are often preterm and of low birth weight. One or other may lie in a difficult position. The second baby may be high, so that a loop of cord can come down before the baby's presenting part has descended. Both babies may need intensive care for the first days or weeks of their lives.

Having said this, I had my own twins at home. I was healthy, with only mild hypertension, the pregnancy went to term, the babies were known to be a good weight and were both head down, and I had an experienced midwife and a supportive partner. These are all important factors that have to be considered.

Labour was brief: they were both born in 90 minutes, one 10 minutes after the other. If I had made the journey to hospital, they would probably have been born in the car. I am glad that I weighed the risks and benefits of going to hospital and made the decision to stay at home, though I remained flexible about switching to hospital if labour was not going well, or if the babies were not in good condition. I had to make the decision without my midwife. When she arrived, she advised me to go to hospital. I asked her to examine me first. She found that the head of the first baby was already on the perineum. There was then no question of moving.

If you have undiagnosed twins, or a twin labour is too fast to risk getting to hospital:

♦ Warm the room and fill hot-water bottles so that the babies will not become cold. Small babies are quickly chilled.

♦ Stay calm. Breathe with a gentle expiration, as slowly as you can. You are breathing for your babies.

♦ Once in the second stage, take it as gently as possible and avoid both hyperventilating and prolonged breath-holding. Your first baby may cope well with these, but the second baby needs good oxygenation for a while longer.

♦ Choose any comfortable position – preferably an upright one (standing, squatting, kneeling, or half-kneeling, half-squatting). If labour is progressing very rapidly, get on all fours.

♦ When the first baby is born, put her to your breast. The sucking will stimulate further contractions to bring the next baby to birth.

A drug to stimulate uterine contractions (syntometrine) should never be given to the mother before the second twin is born. It results in gripping contractions of the uterus that can sometimes trap the second baby.

After the first baby is born, your midwife clamps and cuts the cord, checks the lie of the second baby and listens to the fetal heart. There is space now to adjust the baby to the best position if the lie needs correcting. If labour has not started again in 15 minutes, the usual practice is to rupture the membranes. But, if the firstborn is already suckling at your breast, this will stimulate further contractions that help the second baby towards birth, and there may then be no need to rupture the membranes artificially.

After the birth you will sweat a lot. Even though you may feel cold and shivery, you are giving out a great deal of heat just after the delivery, so hold both babies against you and snuggle under the bedcovers to keep them and yourself beautifully warm.

how can we help the baby who is slow to breathe?

♦ Babies are enormously adaptable. They can manage with very little oxygen for much longer than an adult. Some babies start to breathe as soon as their heads are born. Most take a few seconds to get going. Some start to breathe, but then breathe fitfully for as long as 20 minutes. It takes time for them to adjust. They need to be kept warm and to be touched.

♦ When the cord is not clamped immediately, and it is pulsating, the baby is still receiving some oxygenated blood straight into her bloodstream. There need be no rush to force her to breathe.

♦ Some babies can't breathe well because the respiratory tract is plugged with sticky mucus. When a baby is born with the mother in an upright position, any mucus drains naturally from the mouth and nose. Newborn babies often sneeze mucus out very effectively, too. If a baby needs help to breathe, the first thing to do is to make sure that the airways are clear. She can be placed on her front with the head lower than the hips, so that mucus drains out, while you, or a helper, gently massage her back.

♦ The baby's mouth can be suctioned gently too, using a mucus extractor. It is important not to stimulate the gag reflex by putting the bulb syringe down her throat.

♦ A baby who has had a difficult transition to life needs warmth. Otherwise she uses up a great deal of energy trying to maintain body heat. Most heat loss is from the head, because it is the biggest part. So she should be wrapped in warmed flannel blankets and her head covered. Sometimes a baby is completely floppy and grey and needs oxygen quickly, either mouth-to-mouth or from a bag-mask. Every midwife or doctor attending a birth should carry resuscitation equipment for the rare situation in which this is needed.

If a baby is just flickering and is starting, but not quite managing, to breathe, it helps to talk to the baby: to say "Hello, baby," "Come on love, come on!" or "You're beautiful!" The result may be that the lungs open wider, breaths are deeper, and respiration is more regular. In intensive care nurseries, where babies are being monitored very carefully, oxygen levels often rise when a baby is stroked and when the mother speaks to her baby.

Babies are more likely to have breathing problems when they are born preterm and the lungs are still immature, or when they are born in a hospital where narcotic drugs, such as pethidine, have been given to the mother in high doses.

In spite of the general assumption that babies are slapped on their bottoms to encourage them to breathe, the vast majority of those who are making a slow transition do not benefit from violent stimulation of this kind. If a baby seems dopey and drugged from pain-killers in the mother's bloodstream, her feet can be tickled and, if necessary, a stimulant drug can also be injected.

In some hospitals in Eastern Europe and the USSR, babies are still put under a cold tap. In most hospitals elsewhere a baby who requires resuscitation is put on a special sloping shelf on her back, a tube is pushed down her throat, she is mechanically ventilated, and then given oxygen by face-mask. Elizabeth Davis says that she has witnessed babies whose condition worsens with this treatment, or who struggle to establish their own rhythms. "I usually find myself saying, 'Somebody touch that baby!' Or I move over and do it myself. Observation and participation has taught me· that touch usually brings swift and dramatic improvement."*

There can be a spiritual element in helping a baby to life. Elizabeth Davis also writes of babies being tired after a long labour with a mother too exhausted to welcome a baby. "You use your heart in moments like these. 'What a gorgeous girl (or boy) you have!' Or to the sibling standing by, 'You have a sister (or brother)!' There is a tangible quality of energy that kindles life and response, pure, strong, and loving, and it's the midwife's job to work with everything she's got to initiate this at the given moment."*

what if I bleed heavily?

It is always alarming to see any blood coming from your vagina during pregnancy, even if it is only a few spots. In late pregnancy you may notice slight bleeding after a vaginal examination, and sometimes after sexual intercourse. This is almost always a sign that the cervix is thin, soft, and vascular, and that it may have started to dilate a little already. Occasionally the bleeding is caused by a cervical polyp that has broken away from its stem. This kind of bleeding stops of its own accord.

The show that often heralds labour is a blood-stained mucus plug, like the start of a period. Labour will probably begin within 24 hours after a show, although sometimes a woman goes as long as a week before contractions start. You may have several shows during labour, each heavier than the one before. This is normal.

Antepartum haemorrhage

Real bleeding is a different matter. A steady flow of blood or continual spotting can mean that the placenta is starting to peel away from the lining of the uterus (placental abruption) or that it is in front of the baby's head (placenta praevia). Let your midwife or doctor know what is happening. They will probably get you into hospital as quickly as they can, as an examination should only be done once everything has been set up for Caesarean section.

Such antepartum haemorrhage may occur wherever a woman decides to have her baby, and is not a risk particularly associated with out-of-hospital birth. It is much more common in women who smoke heavily. But every woman should know the symptoms just in case it happens to her.

Bleeding in the third stage

After the baby is born your uterus continues to contract, although you may not be aware of it. The placenta cannot contract, so it peels away from the lining of the uterus, usually within half an hour of the birth, and slips down into your vagina. When this happens and the placenta is ready to be expelled, some bright-red blood appears and the cord lengthens.

The third stage of labour, the time from the birth of the baby until the delivery of the placenta, can be conducted in two ways:

♦ Active management entails an injection of syntometrine – usually into the mother's thigh – as the baby is born, early cord clamping, and immediate removal of the placenta by cord traction.

♦ Physiological management entails allowing time for the cord to stop pulsating before clamping only the baby's end of the cord, letting blood drain into a bowl from the placental section, keeping the mother upright, and allowing her to deliver the placenta and membranes herself by pushing.

These two methods should never be mixed. To do so is a recipe for a retained placenta and postpartum haemorrhage.

Until the placenta separates from the uterine wall there is no bleeding and, even though the placenta may remain in the uterus for a long time, this is not dangerous. Your midwife may press in above your pubic bone and push upwards towards your navel to see if the cord moves up as the uterus is tipped upwards. If it does, the placenta is still attached and no one should pull on the cord, or it may cause bleeding. In hospitals sometimes an energetic attempt to complete the third stage results in the cord breaking. I have also known of women who have had the uterus pulled right down in this way.

"This delivery was so much exactly what a birth should be like, and it made such a strong impression and has given me such an 'easy', confident person of a baby, that I shall always be grateful... It wasn't an earth-shattering experience but almost the opposite – a simple, straightforward event that happened naturally as part of the rhythm of the day."

The partner of a woman who gave birth without assistance phoned me to announce a happy birth three hours before and asked, "When should we expect the placenta?" I advised him to call a midwife, which he declined to do because the local health authority had refused to allow them a home birth. So I suggested that he help his wife into an upright position and, if the placenta did not fall out, that she should remain kneeling and put her lips around the stem of a bottle and give a long blow into it. She did this and the placenta dropped out. There is a traditional practice in South America to free a retained placenta. As air is exhaled, the abdominal press comes into play so that the mother's abdominal muscles press on her fundus and propel the placenta down. This is far safer than heaving the uterus around manually or tugging on the cord.

Postpartum haemorrhage

Occasionally a placenta does not peel away completely, and blood seeps from gaping sinuses in the muscle wall of the uterus. This is postpartum haemorrhage. It is more likely to occur after the uterus has been stretched with twins or with excess amniotic fluid, when a woman has haemorrhaged with a previous birth, following a difficult labour, or where there has been "fundus fiddling" by an anxious attendant. Elizabeth Davis says: "Left to itself the uterus will clamp down uniformly and will sheer off the placenta in one smooth sweep. But if poked and prodded may only release in certain sections."*

With postpartum haemorrhage the mother's blood pressure drops. Especially in poor countries, many women are anaemic and cannot afford a heavy blood loss. Elizabeth Davis recommends a woman in poor health in late pregnancy should have supplementary B vitamins

(100 mg daily), plenty of protein- and iron-rich foods, and alfalfa tablets. Alfalfa is rich in vitamin K which facilitates blood clotting.*

The first thing for the midwife to do if there are signs of haemorrhage is to give an intravenous injection of syntometrine and, if necessary, press the uterus firmly between two hands. A woman bleeds only if her uterus is soft and spongy and does not contract. It should be firm to the touch. If it is not, someone should massage it to stimulate it to contract. You can do this yourself, pressing in as if you are squeezing meringue mixture through an icing nozzle. Nipple stimulation, either from the baby breastfeeding, or manually, also keeps the uterus firm. Once the uterus is firm and contracting, adopt a squatting or all-fours position, and the placenta should be delivered by steady, controlled cord traction with you in this position.

When the placenta is delivered, your midwife will check your pulse and blood pressure and may ask you to continue massaging the uterus to keep it well-contracted. She will stay with you for the next two hours or so.

Nowadays a healthy woman with high haemoglobin in pregnancy can cope with blood loss without having reduced haemoglobin afterwards. All the same, after a bleed it is sensible to take supplementary iron, and to eat iron-rich foods such as chocolate, eggs, molasses, dried fruits, watercress, and other green leafy vegetables. A blood test will be done a few days later to check your haemoglobin level.

The sudden dash to hospital, sirens screaming; the grey and floppy baby who is barely breathing; the woman haemorrhaging massively – these fears are in the back of all our minds. But, because labour out of hospital does not suffer the aggressive intervention to which many hospital labours are subjected, these are extremely rare events.

There is no single ideal birth. There is instead the birth you have, the experience that is uniquely yours. With the support of friends who are sensitive to your needs, quick to respond to your wishes and nurture you, and who above all believe in you and your ability to give birth, childbirth can be an adventure in physical sensation and intense emotion, a journey of discovery of your own inner power that is exhilarating, sensuous and satisfying.

A carefully planned and lovingly conducted home birth, in which the rhythms of nature are respected by a midwife with knowledge and understanding to support the spontaneous unfolding of life, is the safest kind of birth there is.

babymoon

The time immediately following birth is precious. It should never deteriorate to being merely a sequel to delivery, an interval for postpartum recovery, or the kind of "bonding" time in which you feel you must fall in love with the baby fast or you are being an inadequate mother. In birth we have the opportunity ourselves to be reborn, to see the world with new clarity, and to experience life with an intensity that may otherwise be forgotten. A child is born, and for a moment the wheeling planets seem to stop in their tracks, as past, present and future meet. This sense of the miraculous, of incarnation and transcendence, often floods in wherever a baby is born. But when a woman is in her own space, when a couple feel at home in the environment in which they meet this new life, there is a special radiance. Being in a place that you control yourselves means that you need not conform to any standards, be selfconsciously on your best behaviour, or worry about what other people are thinking of you. Instead, you are free to focus entirely on the baby.

planning your babymoon

The babymoon is the old "confinement" in contemporary idiom, adapted to the needs of a woman who, instead of having an extended family, experiences the deepest closeness with her sexual partner. It is a special time in the growth of love, and for many couples has a significance greater than that of the honeymoon, with consequences that may be long-lasting. The idea is simply that the couple create a setting in which they are intimately alone with their baby, and can get to know her without the intrusion of the usual responsibilities and social contacts. Your midwife calls in each day at first, to check on you and the baby, but otherwise you limit other people to a set visiting time, so that your intimacy is not invaded. All the baby-admiring and cuddling and cups of tea and sips of champagne can take place with friends and relatives sitting on and around the bed. At other times you have a note on the door that reads: "Please do not disturb. Family resting."

> "Our neighbours had noticed the comings and goings of the midwives' cars, so my father put up a notice in the window on pink card announcing Grace's arrival. The whole episode became a social event rather than a medical occasion. We plied the midwives with champagne, forgetting they'd missed their lunch, and sent them reeling on their way about six o'clock."

Unless you already have a child, and would welcome someone close to you who can give extra attention to the other child while you get to know your baby, this means putting off having your mother to stay, for example, till the end of this week or ten days, or however long you want the babymoon to last. It also entails careful planning ahead so that your partner can take time off work and you have food in store. If you have a freezer, you can shop and cook well ahead of time. Even if you don't, ensure that the cupboards are full. Before you start labour, buy plenty of fruit juices and other drinks, since breastfeeding makes you thirsty.

Your partner will have to be chef, housekeeper, and butler, unless you rely entirely on take-away meals and let the dishes pile up. The phone is bound to ring a lot. Work out together how you want to deal with that. As well as time to cuddle, you will want time to sleep.

lying in

Traditionally women have always had a "lying in" time, a period of seclusion in which they could concentrate on the new baby and be cared for by other women. Although in situations of extreme poverty, war or famine, it is impossible to ensure this, it remains the ritual ideal in many cultures, and is a powerful functional bond in women's domestic culture.* The 40 days after birth are a time when the new mother is exempt from at least some of her usual tasks, and she receives special consideration, nourishing foods, and loving support from other women of the household, as she passes over the bridge into motherhood. Many of these women stay in the new mother's home for days or weeks afterwards.*

During the earliest part of this period she is in an enclosed space, sometimes a darkened room, and access to outsiders is severely restricted. For she is in a marginal social and spiritual state, and she and the baby are considered to be especially vulnerable and tender.

Within traditional Judaic culture the new mother was cared for entirely by other women for the first 30 days after birth. They built a fire by her and this was fed even on the Sabbath, when such work was normally forbidden, and she was plied with sugary teas and nourishing food.

Usually the time of intensive loving care is shorter than this. In Fiji, for example, the new mother is tended by both of the grandmothers with two young women from her own kin group and two from the father's until the tenth day. In all traditional cultures there are nurturing women to help care for the new baby, take over household tasks such as cleaning and washing, and perhaps massage both mother and baby. They pride themselves on producing especially sustaining foods. In parts of India, for example, they prepare a drink of sweet coconut milk mixed with dill seed, which is thought to give the mother strength.

"It was well after two o'clock on Christmas morning. It was slightly snowing outside and Naomi was peacefully nursing at my breast. We celebrated for another couple of hours before everybody left to get ready for their Christmas celebrations at home."

In today's industrial society, women are often expected to take over cooking and cleaning and caring for their husbands and other children, and to demonstrate that they have "got their figures back", within a few weeks, and sometimes mere days, after birth. They want to return to "normal", as if nothing has happened. It is all supposed to take place without a second thought, and with tremendous joie de vivre. Yet if a new mother is to be able to nurture her child, she needs to be nurtured. Most women need space and time, and cherishing from those closest to them, to make the major adjustment to motherhood, and the focus should be on neither recovery nor return, but on transformation.

"This is when birth at home is so wonderful. You can sleep if and when you want, have the light on to look at your baby when you want, eat and drink when you want. Your husband and children are with you, and everybody can feel uninhibited in greeting and responding to the new baby at their own pace."

If you are having your baby at home, or if you are returning home soon after the birth – the usual arrangement if you have your baby in a birth centre – my suggestion is that you may enjoy postpartum "nesting" in a king-sized bed. The whole focus of the home switches to the bed with its new life. It is as if, for a short space, your bed becomes the household shrine.

welcoming your baby

When a woman first meets her baby, she says goodbye to the fantasy baby inside her and greets the real one in her arms. This can be a difficult transition for a woman who had a clear idea that the baby was of one sex and it turns out to be of the other, or who

"I couldn't help grieving a little. It felt so magical to have her inside me. I had a feeling of emptiness when she was born. She was beautiful, but different from how I had imagined."

was sure that the baby would be perfectly formed and a handicap is revealed, or who expected that the baby would look like her or her partner, or be smaller or larger, or more attractive, than it actually is. A woman strives to find continuity of experience between the baby inside and the baby outside her body. It is not just that she needs time to come to terms with this reality. She may also need a sanctuary in which she can experience safely a range of conflicting

"I knew instantly that she was mine. But there was an odd detachment too. It was as if there were two babies, and the baby inside me was retreating from me while Imogen was coming towards me. Part of me mourned that dark, mysterious baby inside me. At the same time I looked at Imogen and thought, 'We've arrived! Here is my family. Now this house is full of children, and that's how I want it to be.'"

emotions. A hospital is a difficult place in which to do this, with all its comings and goings, the routines of a large institution, and the social isolation from those closest to her that is often imposed on the new mother while she remains a "patient".

For many women who have their babies in hospital bonding is delayed and hindered, or sometimes never gets going, until after they are home, and occasionally not even then. New mothers tell of the frustration, demoralization, and depression at feeling caught up in an alien and threatening system that they are powerless to influence in any way, either for themselves or for their babies. They say such things as: "The nurses were liable to take the babies away with no explanation, and were surprised when asked what they were about to do"; "I felt like one of the cogs in a machine, not a person at all"; and "The mothers seemed to be there for them, and not the other way round."

Hospital staff may consider that the new mother's prime need is for rest, and want to ensure that each woman has uninterrupted sleep at night and rest-times during the day apart from her baby. In some hospitals, for example, babies born at night tend to be sent to the special care nursery even though they are perfectly all right, because it is the easiest thing to do, and it avoids disturbing other mothers.

One result of awareness of the importance of bonding, and of failure to bond being viewed as a cause of child abuse, is that in some hospitals nurses are on the look-out for potential child abusers. Sometimes mothers are acutely aware that they are under critical observation to reveal if they are responding appropriately to their babies. One woman, whose baby suffered from facial palsy, said, "They thought I was in danger of rejecting the baby," and she felt

"I felt my whole body and consciousness expand and fill with pleasure. At that moment I felt that I had been the agent of a miracle, had brought about a revelation not of a truth, but of a life, and with it immense humility and gratitude."

that they thrust him at her. Every time she went to the special care baby unit she felt that she had to put on a performance, and so began to avoid visiting it. The staff's enthusiasm to promote bonding actually made it more difficult for this woman to accept her baby.

Only in a warm, loving, and intimate environment can a woman feel secure in expressing her real emotions. Mothering grows from genuine feelings and bears no resemblance to the magazine image of a glamorous mother in a frilly negligee proudly cradling her new baby. When a woman becomes a mother, she may be swept along as if on a roller-coaster of fierce, passionate, and often conflicting emotions. Her identity as the mother of this particular child is forged not only through pleasure in her baby, but also through the anxiety, pain, and other negative feelings which stem naturally from the "primary maternal preoccupation" that is a normal accompaniment to falling in love with a baby.*

To carry a child in your body, to plan ahead, to make choices between alternatives, to give birth and hold your child in your arms is an experience that can bring with it profound emotional commitment, deep acceptance of responsibility, and a maturing of personality. It is not a medical event. It is a major life transition.

When you greet your baby on your own territory, those who help you come as guests, not guardians of medical space. The whole obstetric system is designed to control women, to render them passive, and to screen, treat, and regulate their reproductive functions for their own good. But in your own personal space there are no rules to be obeyed, no standards to which you must conform. You are free to be yourself.

> "My other two children saw her within minutes. For them birth is a normal process which can happen in the next bedroom, not a dark technological mystery."

Lying together in bed with your baby, you and your partner both have extended time to explore the astonishing reality and the wonder of this new little being. You relive the experience of birth, learn how to respond to his signals, and can start breastfeeding at your own pace and in your own way. Your older children may enjoy cuddling in with you for some of the time, and at other times will need a loving person who can focus on their needs and enable you to have this special time with your baby.

You feel her plump firmness in your arms, stroke the down on the head, and see bright eyes gazing up at you. There is an excitement about breastfeeding that is going well. It is partly the conviction that "your body is working well", and you can both give life and sustain it; partly the sensual physical contact and pleasurable holding and the surge of the milk flow, and partly the pre-verbal conversation with this small human being in your arms, as you get to know a wide-eyed creature for whom the whole world is new, who comes to you out of its raw, elemental being and turns to you in trust.

You will both become aware of your baby's rhythms, the cycles of sleep and waking, the times when he is alert, other times when he is fretful or drowsy, and the highpoints of his life, when he wakes hungry and discovers the firm sweetness of his mother's breasts and sucks avidly until he falls asleep, replete and utterly satisfied. You will enjoy "conversations" with your baby when he is in an awake and alert state. A baby is not merely at the receiving end of stimuli. He can communicate with you by his attention, the steady gaze of his eyes, his restlessness, or the glazed expression that comes on his face before he falls asleep at last. Parents don't need code books to understand this. All they require is unhurried time with their baby in an environment where they can act with spontaneity and are not inhibited by anybody else's expectations or theories. It is an environment that hospitals find very difficult to provide. But it exists already. It is home.

emotional transformation

There is emotional work to be done too. The change from woman to mother occurs as if by grace, by enchantment, but it is also fraught with pain. When you have a baby, your view of the world changes. You see people, and other people's children, with new eyes. You become more vulnerable, more touched by suffering, more sensitively aware of need. You may weep more readily, be distressed by items on news programmes, feel bonded not only with your baby, but with all human beings, all living things, in a different way. Your whole relationship with time changes, and is moulded around your child's need of you. You often feel that time stretches out endlessly like a long ribbon with no end in sight. However it is for you, you cannot go on as before. Life has a new shape.

An older sister:

"It was good that my mum had the baby in the holidays because I was so excited that I did not get to sleep until three o'clock in the morning. For a whole week we had dinner in my mum's room with champagne. Like a picnic to celebrate."

The transformation of woman to mother often has to occur in isolation from that of man to father, and as a result is qualitatively entirely different. After they have a child, many couples find that they each speak a different language and have widely divergent concerns. The mother is child-focused. The father is work-focused. This often happens even when the woman has a career, and up until now has had work at the centre of her life. A man may see a new baby as a possession, but for a woman the child is her flesh. Thus her identity is changed fundamentally, while his is not. You both need a space in your lives to pass through the transformation into being parents, to adjust together to the nakedness of feelings, the new fluidity of time, and the new centre to your lives.

your other children

If you already have a child, this oasis in time is one that nurtures your older child too. She also has to pass through a transformation, from special and only one to older sister, from baby to child. This process of growth cannot be rushed. She, too, needs time and a sanctuary. If your bed is big enough, she can cuddle up with you and the new baby, assured of your love for her, able to get to know the baby in her own way. Keep special playthings and story books close by, and have some favourite snacks handy. She won't want to stay with you long, but will bounce off to play, make things, have an adventure. Your partner will be kept busy coping with your older child's needs as well as yours. This kind of babymoon has a different flavour!

starting to breastfeed

Women can breastfeed against amazing odds. I have been in hospitals in the USSR where mothers are not handed their babies until four hours or longer after birth, by which time nurses have already swaddled them, and where women must have their fingers painted with iodine before they can touch their babies. Yet they breastfeed successfully – because they know they can, and the alternative of artificial feeding is not readily available.

Breastfeeding in hospital

The average hospital environment provides the worst possible start for breastfeeding. In spite of all the lip-service paid to breastfeeding in Britain, for example, in 30 per cent of big hospitals with consultant units women still cannot as a matter of course put their babies to the breast at birth. In 40 per cent babies do not "room-in" with their mothers all the time, and 16 per cent of hospitals allow babies to be with their mothers only in the day-time.*

Babies may be separated from their mothers "so that you can rest," "so that the baby isn't over-stimulated," "so as not to disturb the other mothers," "so that we can keep an eye on him," "because there is a rule that the baby must be in the nursery for the first

Breastfeeding

Q A Will feeding help me bond with my baby?

Yes. Breastfeeding is a natural element in your developing relationship that is exciting and satisfying for you both, an adventure in sensation and touch, and in the gradual unfolding personality of this new human being. Because this is so, it is never merely a matter of technique. It is a way of communicating and loving.

Q A Does breastfeeding hurt?

There may be pain mixed strangely with the tenderness and desire. Your baby's sucking stimulates contractions of the uterus, helping it to return almost to its pre-pregnant size and shape. Your breasts become full, heavy, swollen and tender. When the baby latches on, you feel the urgency of the milk-ejection reflex, and your breasts get flushed, hot and tingling. Make sure that the baby is well latched on, with a good mouthful of breast, or your nipples will become sore and painful, and may even bleed.

Q A Why is breastfeeding important for me?

In addition to the advantages for the baby, breastfeeding is not just a matter of what you do with your breasts, but your sense of positive identity as a woman and a mother. An intense flow of energy surges through your whole body. There is also evidence that it reduces the risk of breast cancer, too.

Q A Is there an advantage in beginning breast-feeding at home?

Yes. It is usually easier to establish breastfeeding at home. The joy of starting to breastfeed in your own environment is that you do not have to put on a demonstration or prove to your carers that you can do it successfully. Instead, it is a secret and delightful conspiracy between you and the baby.

two nights, and your milk hasn't come in, so there is no point in having him with you," or "because the baby is slightly jaundiced and needs phototherapy."

Hospitals are noisy places and in some sedatives are given routinely at night to all mothers, including those who are breastfeeding. One woman commented, "Going without a sleeping tablet seems to be regarded as a perversion." Crying babies are often whisked away to the nursery, and may be given formula by nurses who try to keep the ward peaceful, and who may also enjoy the chance to feed and look after the babies.

Only 30 per cent of hospitals give no additional fluids to breastfed babies: 25 per cent offer water if they think the baby needs it, 7 per cent offer it routinely, and 38 per cent give the babies glucose solution and/or artificial milk. *

A father:

"Ally was very tired after the birth but, because she was at home, she could rest. If she had been forced to adapt to a hospital routine, I think she would have been utterly exhausted."

Women are the target of a great deal of conflicting advice from different caregivers too. They often feel that they have to show that they are following the advice given by whoever is watching them at the time, and as a result become bewildered and disheartened. They sometimes comment that although usually capable and self-assured, they seemed especially vulnerable in hospital, and were surprised at how easily they felt put down or humiliated.

Things are improving now and there is general approval of "demand feeding". Yet even within the same hospital, there may be different interpretations of what this actually is. Many nurses see it as feeding whenever the baby cries, but not more often than every two hours or less than every five hours. In some hospitals mothers are encouraged to follow their babies' lead but must fill in forms indicating when they have fed. It is difficult to do this in a relaxed and spontaneous way because, as one said, "I felt inhibited about owning up to each nibble of colostrum." So they "cheat" on the charts, and give the impression that the baby is suckling less often than is the case.*

"I was given Hilary almost immediately while they dealt with the placenta. She suckled straight away. She was beautiful. When everyone had left and she had been put in her crib, she wouldn't settle, so I lifted her out and I lay nursing her for the rest of the night. Neither Duncan nor I had experienced such complete happiness ever before."

Regulations to keep other staff members happy, including doctors, ward cleaners and caterers, or to present the ward as an orderly, well-managed place to visitors, sometimes restrict feeding-times to certain hours. So mothers may be told that they must not feed at meal-times, during ward cleaning, at rest-times, during the physiotherapy exercise session, during doctors' ward rounds, when they should be having a bath, and at visiting times. As one woman said, "The hospital seemed to treat babies' feeding-times as a necessary evil interrupting hospital routine." As a result babies cry a lot. An Asian mother in a London hospital, wondering at the strange way in which Europeans seem to treat their babies, asked, "Why do the English punish their babies?"

The most usual reasons that are cited for giving up breastfeeding are "insufficient milk", that the baby "rejected the breast or failed to latch on", and "sore nipples".*

Some nurses approve of breastfeeding if it comes easily, but expect mothers to switch to artificial feeding if there are problems, and to stay relaxed about it. They often give tireless devotion, sitting with women to help them establish breastfeeding, but some do not understand the skills of breastfeeding and the art of encouraging a baby to latch on. They are also concerned that emphasis on breastfeeding makes those mothers who are advised to feed artificially feel that they are failures, and seem to hope for a slightly detached attitude in the mother. One woman who resisted the suggestion that her baby should be artificially fed wrote, "The nurse said she had expected trouble with me because I was 'one of those mothers who are determined to breastfeed, come what may'."

It is not surprising that in Britain 19 per cent of first-time mothers and 15 per cent of all mothers have stopped breastfeeding before they leave hospital, and that by the end of the sixth week only 38 per cent are still breastfeeding, and at four months only 26 per cent.* Nearly half of all breastfed babies have artificial milk supplements within their first week of life. By the end of the second week 28 per cent of those babies who had supplementary feeds are fed artificially, compared with 8 per cent of those who had no supplementary feeds.

night nesting

Even after your babymoon has finished, you can keep the same closeness if you have "night nesting". By this I mean that you have your baby sleeping in bed with you instead of in a cot. Traditionally mothers have always slept with their babies, and continue to do so in many cultures, even in the highly evolved industrial society of Japan. In contrast, Western emphasis on children's development of autonomy – being independent and achieving – dictates that a baby should be in his own cot, in his own room, and should not disrupt any adult activities.

When you have your baby in bed with you, the physical closeness, the sounds of your breathing and beating heart, and the warmth of your body are comforting for your baby, and having the baby beside you to touch and to gaze at when you wish is reassuring for you. However busy and rushed you are during the day, night nesting ensures undisturbed time with your baby. You can breastfeed without really waking, and snuggle down with your baby falling asleep again still on your breast.

This is not dangerous. Healthy newborns move their heads away if their noses are obstructed, and are in no danger of being "overlaid", although it is wise not to have a baby in bed if either you or your partner have been drinking heavily or taken drugs that reduce awareness. A really large bed with a firm mattress makes this arrangement more comfortable for all of you. However, there is also an advantage in accustoming the baby to sleeping separately sometimes too, so that later on you do not always have to go to bed every time you want your child to settle down.

"Demand feeding was easy because I had the baby in bed with me."

If you are going back to work again soon after the birth, night nesting and breastfeeding whenever your baby wants to stimulates milk production, and means that you can continue breastfeeding even if your baby is being cared for by someone else for the major part of the day. You may have such a good milk supply that you need to express milk while you are at work lest you become engorged. You can do this simply with a small, portable electric pump, or even by hand if you are adept at it. Then you can store this milk in a refrigerator so that someone else can give it to the baby in a bottle.*

All over the world, in widely varying cultures, women breastfeed while at the same time working in and outside their homes, labouring in the fields, cracking stones to make roads, washing the family's clothing in the river, or gathering berries and other foods in the bush. It is part of a busy life in which the baby's needs are met and the baby is breastfed wherever the mother happens to be. At night mother and baby cuddle in bed together, and the baby may suck on and off through the hours of darkness. This is a pattern of breastfeeding which works well, and one that women in industrial societies are now rediscovering for themselves.

emotions after birth

Nobody knows how many women are unhappy after childbirth. In Western countries one in ten new mothers receives medical treatment for depression.* Almost half of those treated are still depressed a year later. But this is just the tip of the iceberg. Many women do not realize that they are depressed, and many of those who do have no help in dealing with their depression. New mothers often seek advice about breastfeeding difficulties, for example, yet are really asking for help with their own inturned anger and feelings of helplessness and worthlessness. Statistics of clinical depression do not include these distressed women.

Postnatal depression

Postnatal depression is often envisaged as a kind of mental fog that seeps out of a woman's bloodstream and reproductive organs. According to this view, nothing can be done to prevent it, and when it happens women are treated as if they are sick, may be prescribed mood-changing drugs, and be told that ultimately the cure lies within themselves. But, in fact, depression has specific social causes, and there may be many things in a woman's life that contribute to it.

Depression after the birth of a baby is less to do with the hormonal disturbance to which it is often attributed than to all the pressures on a woman to conform to the pattern of a happy new mother, to the socioeconomic stresses on women who are living in poverty,* and, very often, to the experience of being disempowered by childbirth in hospital. My own research reveals that the institutional violence typical of care in many hospitals results in the depersonalization and disabling of women. As a result, some new mothers are left trying to cope with feelings that are very similar to those a woman experiences after being raped, and which often persist weeks, months, and even years later.

There is debate among psychologists and sociologists as to whether obstetric intervention in childbirth is associated with depression. Some research suggests that the more obstetric intervention takes place, the more women suffer from depression.* Women are more likely to be distressed after Caesarean section.* But this may not be depression.

Women who feel that they were denied any control over what was done to them in childbirth are at greater risk of being unhappy in the week following birth than those who feel that they were in control.* This is different from depression, though it may turn into depression. It is post-traumatic stress disorder (PTSD), emotional distress which men, too, may suffer after traumatic events in which they were powerless.* It is not so much whether there is intervention, but a woman's sense of control or loss of control over what is being done to her, that is important.* This may be why women who have planned Caesarean sections are less likely to suffer postnatal depression than those who have unplanned Caesarean sections, when the decision is made once labour has started, often over their heads and over their supine bodies.*

Women who have PTSD after a first baby sometimes decide to have the next birth at home because they are convinced that the hospital environment was in large measure responsible for their later emotional distress. There is mounting evidence that they are right, and that a woman's feelings of wellbeing are enhanced when she is able to give birth in an environment that she herself controls. When you give birth in an environment of your own making – one that you yourself control – you are more likely to experience postnatal euphoria than depression, anxiety or panic.

I am not claiming that if you have your baby at home you will never feel unhappy or unable to cope. But pervading anxiety, panic attacks, loss of confidence, feelings of worthlessness, and an uneasy sense that the baby does not really belong to you and that you have no right to be a mother, are for many women a result of the way in which they are treated when they give birth in hospital. The disempowering of women during a major life transition is distressing not only at the time; it may have long-term emotional effects. The memory of an unhappy birth experience affects a woman's attitude to future pregnancies and may remain with her for many years.

A woman who controls the space in which she gives birth, and who can therefore risk losing her self-control, and surrender to the feelings welling up inside her during birth, is more likely to look back on the birth as a positive experience, and is less vulnerable to depression than one whose autonomy has been destroyed, and who feels that she has been violated.

In an intimate, loving environment, birth can be empowering. Especially for any woman who is vulnerable to depression or violent mood swings, one with low self-esteem, or who has suffered sexual abuse, birth can be healing. Childbirth is then an adventure in which you discover your own inner strength, joy in your body, and your capacity to give life and to open yourself in love.

postscript

Birth, like death, is a human experience we all share. It can be an interruption of life, a medical episode, a solitary trial of endurance, an operation on a patient who relies entirely on obstetric expertise, and a frightening process in which women are trapped by their biology. Or it can be lived through in beauty and dignity, as new life emerges cradled in love and caring, it can be a celebration which takes place in spite of pain. For the energy flooding through a woman's body in birth, although it brings pain, is life-enhancing and powerful.

Choosing their birthplace – in which they feel secure – creating a nest that meets the needs of mother and newborn, is something all mammals do, unless, like animals in a zoo, they are in captivity.

Women in our post-industrial culture are effectively captive in birth. The zoo may be run on scientific principles, the keepers may be considerate and may pride themselves on the good condition of their animals and the low mortality rate. Visiting times may be frequent and the zoo may be friendly and welcoming. In the cage there may be space to move about, and those in charge may have tried to replicate the natural habitat. Yet captivity restrains and dictates the behaviour of the captives.

At present saying "no" to birth in a hospital environment, making an informed decision to give birth in a place of your choosing, is for most of us the only way to reclaim the experience of birth for women. There is a challenge facing the maternity services today over and above the basic requirement to make birth as safe as possible for mothers and babies. This challenge consists of two main issues. The first is to provide genuine choice. It must include the provision of a really good home birth service and, for those who prefer them, small GP units and alternative birth centres. The second important issue is to enable women giving birth in hospital to control the birthplace there, too, so that they are not merely at the receiving end of care, however kind and compassionate it may be.

When we affirm our freedom by making an informed choice, and select a place where we, not the doctors, are in control, we have an opportunity to rediscover in ourselves the power to give birth without intervention, with the confidence and spontaneity with which we breathe and move, and with the same love and passion with which we may have conceived the child who enters the world.

useful addresses

Birth Classes
Active Birth Centre
25 Bickerton Road,
London N19 5JT
020 7482 5554
www.activebirthcentre.
com

National Childbirth Trust
020 8992 8637
www.nctpregnancyandbaby
care.com

Irish Childbirth Trust
001 8724501

Water Birth: Pools
Aqua Pool Hire
01425 616734

Blue Lagoon
01695 556642

Beacon House
Woodley Park,
Skelmersdale,
Lancashire WN8 6UR

Splashdown
020 8422 9308
www.waterbirth.co.uk

See also Active Birth Centre

See "Midwifery Guidelines
on the Use of Water" by
Ethel Burns and
Sheila Kitzinger
Eburns@brookes.oc.uk

Acupuncture
British Acupuncture
Council
020 8735 0400
www.acupuncture.
org.uk

Alexander Technique
Society of Teachers of
the Alexander Technique
020 7284 3338
birth: 020 8969 5356
www.stat.org.uk

**Awarness Through
Movement**
Feldenkrais Guild UK
P.Obox 370,
London N10 3XA
Freephone 07000 785 506
Enquiries@feldenkrais.co.uk
www.feldenkrais.co.uk.

Antenatal Tests
Support during antenatal
testing 020 7631 0285

Aromatherapy
International Federation
of Aromatherapists:
020 8742 2605
www. Int-fed-aromatherapy.
co.uk

Birth Centres
Birth Centre Network
020 7476 1977,
www.birthcentres@yahoo
groups.com

Breastfeeding
La Leche League
020 7242 1278

National Childbirth Trust
Breastfeeding Line
0870 444 8708.

Breastfeeding Network
0800 900 8787
PO Box 11126, Paisley
PA2 8YB

Association of
Breastfeeding Mothers
020 7813 1481
PO Box 207,
Bridgwater TA6 7YT

Fatherhood
Families Need Fathers
020 7613 5060

Single Parents
Gingerbread
Support for lone
parents.
0800 0184318,
www.gingerbread.
org.uk

National Council for
One Parent Families
Information on financial,
legal and housing
problems.
0800 0185026,
www.oneparentfamilies.
org.uk

Homeopathy
British Homeopathic
Association
020 7566 7800
www.trusthomeopathy.org

Hypnosis
British Hypnotherapy
Association
020 7723 4443

Midwives
Independent Midwives
Association
01483 358615
www.independentmidwives.
  org.uk

Royal College of
Midwives
020 7312 3535

Association of Radical
Midwives
01695 572776

Home Birth
International Home
Birth Movement
01865 300154

Miscarriage
Miscarriage Association
01924 200799
www.miscarriageassociation.
  org.uk

Doulas
Independent Doula
Association
doula.training@virgin.net

Independent Doula
Association of Scotland
14 Cherry Lane,
Cupar, Fife
Scotland KY15 5DA
01334 655 786
doula.training@virgin.net

Millennia Doulas
020 7722 4786
doula@org.uk

Safe Hands Doulas
www.safehands-doulas.co.uk

BOND
British School of
Nurturing Doulas:
020 7274 3968

Hefferlumps
020 8405 3919
hefferlumpsandco@
  another.com

Reflexology
Association of
Reflexologists
0870 5673320
www.aor.org.uk

General Practitioners
Royal College of General
Practitioners
020 7581 3232

Twins
Twins and Multiple Birth
Association (TAMBA)
01732 868000,
www.tamba.org.uk

Caesareans
Caesarean Support
Network
01624 661269

Vaginal Birth After
Caesarean (VBAC)
8 Wren Way,
Farnborough, Hants
GU14 8SZ
01243 868440

Vegetarians
The Vegetarian Society
0161 925 2000,
www.vegsoc.org

Websites
Sheila Kitzinger's Website
www.sheilakitzinger.com

www.homebirth.org.uk

www.babydirectory.com

Further reading
Sheila Kitzinger –
Pregnancy & Childbirth,
Penguin,
Breastfeeding,
Dorling Kindersley

MIDIRS Informed Choice
Leaflets
Freecall 0800 581009
www.midivs.org

references

These research references relate to the asterisks in the main text. Where there is more than one asterisk on a page, the references appear in order, with each entry on a new line relating to a different asterisk.

p.11 Doering S., Entwistle D. (1975) "Preparation during pregnancy and ability to cope with labor and delivery", *American Journal of Orthopsychiatry*, 45, 825–837; Norr K., Block C., Charles A., Meyering S., Meyers F. (1977) "Explaining pain and enjoyment in childbirth", *Journal of Health and Social Behaviour*, 10, 260–275; Doering S., Entwistle D., Quinlan D. (1980) "Modeling the quality of women's birth experience", *Journal of Health and Social Behavior*, 21, 12–21; Entwistle D., Doering S. (1981) *The First Birth*, Baltimore: John Hopkins University Press; Romito P. (1989) "Unhappiness after childbirth", *Effective Care in Pregnancy and Childbirth*, 2, 1433–1446, eds. Chalmers I., Enkin M., Keirse M. J. N. C.; Kitzinger. J. in Garcia J., Kilpatrick R., Richards M. (1990) *The Politics of Maternity*

Care, Oxford: Clarendon Press; Kitzinger S., "Childbirth and violence against women", (forthcoming) *Women's Health Matters*, ed. Roberts H., London: Routledge.
♦ Kitzinger S. (1987) *Some Women's Experiences of Epidurals*, London: National Childbirth Trust.

p.19 Morse J M, Park C, (1988) "Home birth and hospital deliveries: A comparison of the perceived painfulness of parturition", *Research in Nursing & Health*, 11, 175–181
♦ Lowe N. K. (1987) "Individual variation in childbirth pain", *Journal of Psychosomatic Research* 20, 212–221, Fridh G, Kopare T, Gaston-Jophansson F, Turnell Norvell K, (1988) "Factors associated with more intense labor pain". *Research in Nursing and Health* 11, 117–124)

p.20 Morse J. M., Park C., (1988) "Home birth and hospital deliveries: A comparison of the perceived painfulness of parturition", *Research in Nursing & Health*, 11 175–181, Fridh G, Kopare T, Gaston-Jophansson F, Turnell

Norvell K, (1988) Factors associated with more intense labor pain. *Research in Nursing and Health* 11, 117–124
♦ Fridh G., Kopare T., Gaston-Jophansson F., Turnell Norvell K, (1988) Factors associated with more intense labor pain. *Research in Nursing and Health* 11, 117–124
♦ Simkin P. (1986) "Stress, pain and catecholamines in labor: part 1, a review", *Birth*, 13, 4, 227–233.

p.21 Association of Anaesthetists (1988) *Report on Obstetric Services*, London.

p.22 Geoffrey Chamberlain and Luke Zander, "Induction", *British Medical Journal* 318,1999, 995–997

♦ Kitzinger S. (1975) *Some Women's Experiences of Induced Labour*, London: National Childbirth Trust.

p.25 O'Driscoll K., Meagher D. (1980) "Active management of labour", *Clinical and Obstetric Gynaecology* (supplement 1), ed. W.B. Saunders.
♦ ibid.
♦ ibid.
♦ ibid.

p.26 Taylor R. W., Taylor M. (1988) Letter to the *Lancet* 1, 8581, 352.

♦ Nielson P. V., Stigsby B., Nickelson C., Nim J. (1987) "Intra- and inter-observer variability in the assessment of intrapartum cardiotocograms", *Acta Obstetricia et Gynecologia Scandinovica*, 66, 421–424.

♦ Grant A. (1989) "Monitoring the fetus during labour", *Effective Care in Pregnancy and Childbirth*, 2, 846–882, Oxford: Oxford University Press, eds. Chalmers I., Enkin M., Keirse M. J. N. C.

♦ Macdonald D., Grant A., Sheridan-Pereira M., Boylan P., Chalmers I. (1985) "The Dublin randomized trial of intrapartum fetal heart rate monitoring", *American Journal of Obstetrics and Gynecology*, 152, 524–539.

♦ ibid.; Grant A., (1987b) "The relationship between obstetrically preventable intrapartum asphyxia, abnormal neonatal neurological signs and subsequent motor impairment in babies born at or after term", *Perinatal Events and Brain Damage in Surviving Children*, Berlin: Springer Verlag, eds. Kubli F., Patel N., Schmidt W., Linderkamp O.

p.27 Amato J. G. (1983) "Fetal heart-rate monitoring", *American Journal of Obstetrics and Gynecology*, 147, 967–969.

♦ Visser G. H. A., Goodman J. U. S., Dawes G. 5. (1980) "Problems with ultrasonic fetal heart-rate monitor", *Lancet*, 1, 707–708.

p.28 Sharp D. G., Couriel J. M. (1985) "Penetration of the subarachnoid space by fetal scalp electrode", *British Medical Journal*, 291, 1169.

♦ d'Souza S. W. (1982) "Fetal scalp damage and neonatal jaundice: A risk of fetal scalp electrode monitoring", *International Journal of Obstetrics and Gynecology*, 2, 161–164.

♦ Enkin M. (1989) "Labour and delivery following previous caesarean section", *Effective Care in Pregnancy and Childbirth*, 2, 1196–1217, eds. Chalmers I., Enkin M., Keirse M. J. N. C.

p.30 Inger Findley and Geoffrey Chamberlain "ABC of Labour Care: Relief of Pain", *British Medical Journal* 318, 1999 pp927–930

p.31 Kitzinger S. (1989) "Perceptions of pain in home and hospital birth", Paper given at the International Congress of Psychosomatic Obstetrics and Gynaecology, Amsterdam.

p.32 Garcia J., Garforth S., Ayers S. (1986) "Midwives confined? Labour ward policies and routines", *Research and the Midwife Conference Proceedings*, University of Manchester, 74–78.

♦ Cohen W. R. (1977) "Influence of the duration of second stage labor on perinatal outcome and puerperal morbidity", *Obstetrics and Gynecology*, 49, 266–269.

♦ Caldeyro-Barcia R. (1979) "The influence of maternal bearing-down efforts during second stage on fetal wellbeing", *Birth and the Family Journal*, 6, 17–21.

♦ Thacker S. F., Banta H. D. (1983) "Benefits and risks of episiotomy: An interpretive review of the English language literature, 1860–1980", *Obstetrical and Gynecological Survey*, 38, 322–338.

p.33 ibid.; Sleep J. M., Grant A., Garcia J., Elbourne D., Spencer J., Chalmers I. (1984) "West Berkshire perineal management trial", *British Medical Journal*, 289, 587–590; Harrison R. F., Brennan M., North P. M., Reed J. V., Wickham F. A. (1984) "Is routine episiotomy necessary?", *British Medical Journal*, 288, 1971–1975; Sleep J. M., Grant A. (1987)

"West Berkshire perineal management trail: Three year follow-up", *British Medical Journal*, 295, 749–751.
◆ Sleep J. M., Grant A., Garcia J., Elbourne D., Spencer J., Chalmers I., op. cit.; Harrison R. F., Brennan M., North P. M., Reed J. V., Wickham E. A., op. cit.
◆ Kitzinger S., Simkin P. (1990) *Episiotomy and the Second Stage of Labor*, Pennypress Inc.
◆ Kitzinger S., Walters R. (1981) *Some Women's Experiences of Episiotomy*, London: National Childbirth Trust.

p.34 ibid
◆ ibid
◆ ibid.

p.35 ibid
◆ ibid
◆ Davis E. (1981) *Heart and Hands*, California: Celestial Arts; Flint C. (1988) *Sensitive Midwifery*, London: Heinemann, 101–102.

p.36 Harold Neu, "The crisis in antibiotic resistance". *Science* 257, pp1064–73, 1992

p.37 Cordero L., Hon E. (1971) "Neonatal bradychardia following nasopharyngeal stimulation", *Journal of Pediatrics*, 78, 441–447.
◆ Tyson J., Silverman W., Reisch J. (1989) "Immediate care of the newborn infant", *Effective Care in Pregnancy and Childbirth*, 2,1293–1312, eds. Chalmers I., Enkin M., Keirse M. J. N. C.
◆ ibid.
◆ Cordero L., Hon E., op. cit.; Widstrom A.-M., RansjoArvidson A. B., Christeosson K., Matthieson A-S., Winberg, J., Uvnas-Moberg K. (1987) "Gastric suction in healthy newborn infants: Effect on circulation and developing feeding behaviour", *Acta Paediatrica Scandinavica*, 76, 566–572.
◆ Wahlberg V., Lundh W., Winberg J. (1982b) "Reconsideration of Crede prophylaxis III: Effects of silver nitrate prophylaxis on visual alertness in neonates", *Acta Paediatrica Scandinavica*, 295 (Supplement), 43–48; Wahlberg V., Lundh W., Winberg J. (1982c) "Reconsideration of Crede prophylaxis IV: Effects of silver nitrate prophylaxis on mother infant relationship", *Acta Paediatrica Scandinavica*, 295 (Supplement), 49–57; Wahlberg V., Lundh W., Winberg J. (1982d) "Reconsideration of Crede prophylaxis V: Long-term influences on conjunctival secretion, infant behaviour, breastfeeding and maternal feelings. A descriptive study", *Acta Paediatrica Scandinavica* (Supplement) 59–67.
◆ Rothenberg (1979) "Ophthalmia neonatorum due to Neisseria gonorrhoeae: Prevention and treatment", *Sexually Transmitted Diseases*, 6 (Supplement), 187–190.
◆ Hammerschlag M. R., Chandler J. W., Alexander R., English M., Chiang W. T., Koutsky L., Esehenbach D. A., Smith J. R. (1980) "Erythromycin ointment for ocular prophylaxis of neonatal chlamydial infection", *Journal of the American Medical Association*, 244, 2291–2293.

p.38 World Health Organization (1985).

p.42 Mahmood T A, Campbell D M , Wilson A. W. (1988) "Maternal height, shoe size, and outcome of labour in white primigravidas: A prospective anthropometric study", *British Medical Journal*, 297, 515–517.

p.43 Campbell R., Macfarlane A. (1990) "Recent debate on the place of birth". *The Politics of Maternity Care*, Oxford University Press, 217–237, eds. Garcia J., Kilpatrick R., Richards M.
◆ Social Security Committee (1980) *Perinatal and Neonatal*

Mortality (second report), London: HMSO

p.45 H. C. Woodcock, A. W. Read, D. J. Moore and others "Planned home-births in Western Australia 1981–1987: A descriptive study" *Medical Journal of Australia* 153: pp672–678, 1990)

p.46 Tew M. (1990) *Safer Childbirth*, London: Chapman & Hall
♦ Ole Olsen, "Meta-analysis of the Safety of Home Birth", *Birth* 24:1 March 1997 pp4–13

p.47 Geoffrey Chamberlain, Ann Wraight, Patricia Crowley, "Home Birth: The Report of the 1994 Confidential Enquiry by the National Birthday Trust Fund", Parthenon, London 1997

p.48 Wright J. T. (1983) "Alcohol and drug abuse in pregnancy", *Medicine International*, 35, 1630–1631.
♦ Calandra C., Abell D. A., Beiseher N. A. (1981) "Maternal obesity in pregnancy," *Obstetrics and Gynecology*, 57, 8–12; Garbakiak J. A., Richter M., Miller S., Barton J. J. (1985) "Maternal weight and pregnancy complications", *American Journal of Obstetrics and Gynecology*, 152, 238–245.

♦ Garbakiak J. A. *et al*, op. cit.
♦ Chamberlain R. *et al*, op. cit.; eds. James D. K., Stirrat G. M. (1988) *Pregnancy and Risk: The Basis for Rational Management*, Chichester: John Wiley & Sons.

p.49 Hofmeyr G. J. (1989) "Breech presentation and abnormal lie in late pregnancy", *Effective Care in Pregnancy and Childbirth*, 1, 635–666, Oxford: Oxford University Press, eds. Chalmers I., Enkin M., Keirse M.J. N. C.
♦ Hughey M. J. (1985) "Fetal position during pregnancy", *American Journal of Obstetrics and Gynecology*, 153, 885–886.
♦ Westgren M., Edvall H., Nordstrom F., Svalenius P. (1985) "Spontaneous cephalic version of breech presentation in the late trimester", *British Journal of Obstetrics and Gynaecology*, 92, 19–22.

p.50 Bakketeig L. S., Hoffman H. J. (1981) "Epidemiology of preterm birth: Results from a longitudinal study of births in Norway", Preterm Labour, London: *Butterworth's International Medical Review*, 17–40, eds. Elder M. G., Hendricks C. H.
♦ Salzmann B. (1964) "Rupture of low segment cesarean section", *American*

Journal of Obstetrics and Gynecology, 23, 460–466.
♦ Beard R. W., Lowy C. (1986) "The British survey of diabetic pregnancies", *British Journal of Obstetrics and Gynaecology*, 89, 78326.
♦ James D. K., Stirrat G. M. eds., op. cit., 58.
♦ de Swiet M. (1986) "Preexisting medical diseases", *Prepregnancy Care: A Manual for Practice*, Chichester: John Wiley & Sons, 69–111, eds. Chamberlain G., Lumley J.

p.52 Bird C. (1971) "The premenopausal gravida", *Journal of Reproductive Medicine*, 6, 48–50.
♦ Kirz D. S., Dorchester W., Freeman R. K. (1985) "Advanced maternal age", *American Journal of Obstetrics and Gynecology*, 152, 1, 7–12.
♦ Cario G. M., Fray R. E., Morris N. P. (1985) "The obstetric performance of the elderly primigravida", *British Journal of Obstetrics and Gynoecology*, 54, 237–240.

p.53 Taylor David J. et al (1985) "Do pregnancy complications contribute to neurodevelopmental disability?", *Lancet*, 1, 713–716.

p.54 Steer P. (1988) "Risks in labour", *Pregnancy and Risk*, 6, 105–137, eds. James D. K., Stirrat G. M.

p.61 Dawn Saunders and others, Evaluation of the Edgware Birth Centre, North Thames Perinatal Public Health, London, 2000)

p.66 Feldman E., Hurst M. (1987) "A comparison of hospital and birth center settings", Birth, 18–24.
♦ Lumley J., Davey B. (1987) "Do hospitals with family-centered maternity care policies have lower intervention rates?", *Birth*, 132–134.

p.67 Klein M. *et al* (1984) "Care in a birth room versus a conventional setting: A controlled trial", *Canadian Medical Association Journal*, 131, 1461–1466.
♦ Rosenblatt K. A., Reinken J., Shoemack P. (1985) "Is obstetrics safe in small hospitals? Evidence from New Zealand's regionalized perinatal system", *Lancet*, 2, 429–432.

p.68 Mugford M., Stilwell J. (1986) "Maternity services: how well have they done and could they do better?" *Health Care*, Policy Journals.

p.73 Human Rights Act, Stationery Office, London 1998

p.80 Hood S. (1989) "Midwifery in some European countries", eds. van Hall E. V., Everaerd W., op cit.

p.81 Barrington E. (1985) "Birth stories and midwives' musings", *Midwifery is Catching*, 101.

p.82 Kirkham M. A. (1986) "A feminist perspective in midwifery", *Feminist Practice in Women's Healthcare*, Chichester: John Wiley & Sons, ed. Webb C.

p.90 WHO Regional Office for Europe (1986) adapted from *Having a Baby in Europe*, Copenhagen.

p.91 Serkin M.,Porte J.A., Monheit A. G. (May 1988) "The relationship of antepartum pelvic examinations to the incidence of premature rupture of the membranes, maternal infection, and caesarean section", Paper given at the Scientific Session of Annual Clinical Meeting of American College of Obstetricians and Gynecologists.
♦ Pearce J. M., Campbell S. (1987) "A comparison of symphysis-fundal height and ultrasound as screening tests for light-for-gestational age infants", *British Journal of*

Obstetrics and Gynoecology, 94, 100–104.
♦ Alexander S. *et al* (1989) "Biochemical assessment of fetal well-being", *Effective Care in Pregnancy and Childbirth*, 1, 455–476, eds. Chalmers I., Enkin M, Keirse M J N C
♦ Mohide P., Keirse M. J. N. C. (1989) "Biophysical assessment of fetal well-being", eds. Chalmers I., Enkin M., Keirse M. J. N. C., op. cit., 455–476.

p.89 Office of Population Censuses and Surveys (1986) *Mortality Statistics, Perinatal and Infant: Social and Biological Factors*, Series DH3, London: HMSO, 17.

p.93 Robinson M. (1958) "Salt in pregnancy", *Lancet*, 1, 178–181.
♦ Rush D. (1989) "Effects of changes in protein and calorie intake during pregnancy on the growth of the human fetus", eds. *Chalmers I.*, Enkin M., I. Keirse M. J. N. C., op. cit., 255–280.
♦ ibid.

p.94 McIntyre A. (1988) *Herbs for Pregnancy and Childbirth*, London: Sheldon.

p.95 Hemminki E., Starfield B. (1985) "Routine

administration of iron and vitamins during pregnancy: Review of controlled clinical trials", *British Journal of Obstetrics and Gynaecology*, 85, 404–410.
♦ Alexander S. *et al*, op. cit.

p.115 Ethel Burns and Sheila Kitzinger, "Midwifery Guidelines for Use of Water in Labour", OCRAD, *Oxford Brookes University*, OX3 7PD, 2001

p.118 Richards M., Dunn J., Antonis B. (1977) "Caretaking in the first year of life: The role of fathers' and mothers' social isolation", *Child Care Health Development*, 3, 23–36.

p.120 Berry L. M. (1988) "Realistic expectation of the labor coach", *Journal of Obstetric Gynecologic and Neonatal Nursing*, 17, 5, 354–355.

p.123 Perez P., Snedeker C. (1990) "Why parents need professional labor support", *Special Women*, Pennypress Inc.

p.129 Kitzinger S. (1989) *Pregnancy and Childbirth*, London: Michael Joseph.

p.134 Donnison J. (1990) *Midwives and Medical Men*, London: Heinemann.
♦ Pollock L. (1987) *A Lasting Relationship: Parents and Children*

over Three Centuries, London: Fourth Estate.

p.135 Mason J. (1988) quoting Miles L., "Pioneer Questionnaires (Health) SX-2" in "Midwifery in Canada", *The Midwife Challenge*, London: Pandora, ed. Kitzinger S.
♦ ibid.
♦ Benoit C. (Winter 1983) "Midwives and healers: The Newfoundland experience", *Health Sharing*, 22–25.

p.136 ibid.
♦ Klaus M., Kennell J., Robertson S., Sosa R. (1986) "Effects of social support during parturition on maternal-infant morbidity", *British Medical Journal*, 293, 585–587.

p.137 Hodnett F. D., Osborn R. W. (1989) "A randomized trial of the effects of monitrice support during labor: Mothers' views two to four weeks postpartum", *Birth*, 16, 4, 177–184.

p.138 Flint C. (1986) *Sensitive Midwifery*, London: Heinemann.

p.144 Rossavik 1. K. (1989) *Obstetrics and Gynecology*, 73, 2, 243–249.
♦ PL Yudkin, L Wood and CWG Redman "Rise of

unexplained stillbirth at different gestational ages." *Lancet* pp1192–4, 1987
♦ Lamont R. F. (1986) "Management of preterm labour", *Hospital Update*, 487–490, 492–493.
♦ Salmon Y. M. (1986) "Cervical ripening by breast stimulation", *Obstetrics and Gynecology*, 67, 1, 21–24; Curtis P. (1986) "Uterine responses to three techniques of breast stimulation", *Obstetrics and Gynecology*, 67, 1, 22–28; Curtis F. (1986) "Prepartum and intrapartum breast stimulation in obstetrics", *Journal of Reproductive Medicine*, 31, 4, 228–230.

p.147 Sinquefield G. (1985) "Midwifery management of premature rupture of the membranes at term", *Journal of Nurse Midwifery*, 30, 4, 242–244.
♦ Lenihan J. P. (1984) "The relationship of antepartum pelvic examinations to premature rupture of the membranes", *Obstetrics and Gynecology*, 63, 33–37.

p.149 Davis F. (1987) *Heart and Hands*, California: Celestial Arts.

p.150 Butler N. R., Bonham D.G. (1963) *Perinatal Mortality*, Edinburgh: Churchill Livingstone.

◆ McKay S. (1983) "How worthwhile are membrane stripping and amniotomy?", *Contemporary Obstetrics and Gynecology*, 173–176, 178–181,184.

p.152 Newton N., Foshea D., Newton M. (1966) "Experimental inhibition of labor through environmental disturbance", *Obstetrics and Gynecology*, 67, 371–377.

p.154 Salar G. *et al*, "Effect of transcutaneous electrotherapy on cerebra-spinal fluid beta-endorphin content in patients without pain problems", *Pain*, 10, 169–172; Polden M. (1985) Transcutaneous nerve stimulation in labour and post-Caesarean section", *Physiotherapy*, 71, 8, 350–353.

p.155 Harrison R. F. *et al* (1986) "Pain relief in labour using transcutaneous electrical nerve stimulation (TENS)", *British Journal of Obstetrics and Gynaecology*, 93, 7, 739, 746.

p.156 Flint C., op. cit.
◆ Davis E., op. cit.
◆ Simkin P. (1989) *The Birth Partner*, The Harvard Common Press.

p.158 Gaskin I. M. (1982) "Ask the midwives", *The Practicing Midwife*, 1, 15.

p.161 Lawrence H. (1988) "Breathing for labour", *Journal of Association of Chartered Physiotherapists and Obstetrics in Gynaecology*, 60, 2, 21–23.
◆ Broach J., Newton N. (June 1988) "Food and beverages in labor. Part 1: Cross-cultural and historical practices. Part 2: The effects of cessation of oral intake during labor", *Birth*, 2, 15.
◆ Davis E., op. cit.

p.163 Newton N., Foshea D., Newton M., op. cit.

p.164 J. Sleep, J. Roberts, I. Chalmers, "Care during the second stage of labour", in Murray Enkin, Marc J.N.C. Keirse, James Neilson and Others, *A Guide to Effective Care in Pregnancy and Childbirth*, Oxford University Press, Third Edition, 2000
◆ Cronk M., Flint C. (1989) *Community Midwifery: A Practical Guide*, London: Heinemann.

p.165 Gaskin I. M. (1978) *Spiritual Midwifery*, Tennessee: The Book Publishing Co.

p.166 Stein A. (1986) "Breech delivery: A co-

operative nurse-midwifery medical management approach", *Journal of Nurse-Midwifery*, 31, 2, 93–97.
◆ Odent M. (1984) *Birth Reborn*, New York: Random House.
◆ Russell J. G. B. (1982) "The rationale of primitive delivery positions", *British Journal of Obstetrics and Gynaecology*, 89, 712–715.

p.168 J. Sleep, J. Roberts, I, Chalmers, op.cit

p.169 O'Leary J. A., Gunn D. L. (1986) "Option for shoulder dystocia: cephalic replacement", *Contemporary Obstetrics and Gynecology*, 27, 157.
◆ Gaskin I. M. (1988) "Shoulder dystocia: Controversies in management", *Birth Gazette*, 5, 1, 14–17.
◆ Flint C., op. cit.

p.172 Davis E., op. cit.
◆ ibid.

p.174 ibid.
p.175 ibid

p.178 Leavitt J. W. (1986) *Brought to Bed: Childbearing in America 1750-1950*, New York: Oxford University Press
◆ Sheila Kitzinger, *Rediscovering Birth*, Little Brown, 2000

p.182 Winnicott D. J. (1964) *The Child, the Family, and The Outside World*, London: Penguin.

p.184 Garforth S., Garcia J. (1989) "Breastfeeding policies and practice – 'no wonder they get confused'", *Midwifery*, 5, 2, 75–83.

p.186 ibid.
◆ Kitzinger S. (1983) *The New Good Birth Guide*, London: Penguin, 139–142.

p.187 Woolridge M. W. (1988) "Right from the start – establishing breastfeeding", Symposium on Caring for the Breastfeeding Mother, London: Kings Fund Centre.
◆ Office of Population, Censuses and Surveys, Social Security Division (1988) *Infant feeding* 1985, London: HMSO.

p.188 Kitzinger S. (1988) *Breastfeeding your Baby*, London: Dorling Kindersley.

p.189 Pitt B. (1968) "Atypical depression following childbirth", *British Journal of Psychiatry*, 114,1325–1335,
◆ Stein A. *et al* (1989) "Social adversity and perinatal complications: Their relation to postnatal depression", *British Medical Journal*, 290.
◆ Oakley A. (1980) *Women Confined*, Oxford: Martin Robertson.
◆ Affonso D. (1981) *Impact of Cesarean Childbirth*, Philadelphia: Davis; Bradley C. P. *et al* (1983) "A prospective study of mothers' attitudes and feelings following cesarean and vaginal births", *Birth* 10, 79–83; Garel M. et al (1987) "Psychological consequences of caesarean childbirth in primiparas", *Journal of Psychosomatic Obstetrics and Gynaecology*, 6, 197–209.

p.190 Thune-Larsen K. B., Mailer Pedersen K. (1988) "Childbirth experience and postpartum emotional disturbance", *Journal of Reproductive and Infant Psychology*, 6, 229–240.
◆ Entwistle D, Doering S. (1981) *The First Birth*, Baltimore: John Hopkins University Press; Green J., Coupland V., Kitzinger J. *Great Expectations* (based on research by Child Care Development Group, University of Cambridge), Kitzinger S. (1989) *The Crying Baby*, London: Penguin.
◆ Garel M. *et al*, op. cit.

index

acknowledgements

I should like to thank my many friends and colleagues in the birth movement internationally who have explored with me different aspects of the subject of birth at home and in birth centres. My daughter, Tess Mckenney, who is my website designer and manager, also works with me, giving information and support to women who seek help from the International Home Birth Movement. Rachel Clark, Lorna Munroe and Michele Dodd have provided invaluable secretarial assistance. This book could never have been written without all the women who have discussed with me their own birth experiences, and I have learned a great deal from them. Thank you.

Publisher's acknowledgements
The publishers would like to thank Anna Bedewell for picture research, Jess Hughes, Claire Cross and Michelle Crane for editorial assistance, Liz Brown for design assistance and Hilary Bird for the index.

picture credits

The publisher would like to thank the following for
their kind permission to reproduce their photographs:
(Abbreviations key: t=top, b=bottom, r=right, l=left, c=centre)
Bubbles: Franz Rombout 142.
Corbis Stock Market: LWA-Dann Tardiff 132.
Family Life Picture Library/Angela Hampton: 4, 86, 112, 116.
Sally & Richard Greenhill: 176.
Mother & Baby Picture Library/emap esprit: Ruth Jenkinson 2.
Science Photo Library: Ruth Jenkinson 76.
The Wellcome Institute Library, London: Anthea Sieveking 12, 58.
Uwe Kitzinger: 40

Jacket picture credits
Front jacket: Photonica: Ann Cutting
Inside flap: Newsquest

All other images Marcia May © Dorling Kindersley.
For further information see: www.dkimages.com